Who
al
Conflicts

CW00853058

Mark Aitken

ISBN : 9798403160872

Dedication

This book is dedicated to everyone who has given their undivided support to our National Health Service, without expecting anything in return, and to those in today's vanguard who are determined to pursue the ideals of Aneurin (Nye) Bevan's original dream.

I also want to make a special mention for those working in charitable institutions like the MacMillan Nurses in our hospices, and in particular the St Helena Hospice in Colchester to which the Royalties from this book will be donated.

Caring for someone for whom there is no hope of recovery, and where the sole aim and object of the carer is to make the last few days of life free from the mental and physical agony of the underlying disease, doesn't bring the same sense of achievement which comes with having nursed a sick patient back to health. So, these carers are really special.

We sometimes glibly talk about allowing a terminally ill patient to die at home as being the most caring option, but we forget that the experience for the spouse could be a nightmare, because once the patient has died, there are the awful tasks of getting a doctor to certify the death, and getting the undertakers to remove the body.

When patients die they rarely die with a smile on their lips!

MacMillan Nurses protect the living from witnessing the death throes of their nearest and dearest, so that the memories which survive are those of happier times.

Contents

PART FIVE
Dismembering the NHS Carcase

PART SIX
Public Involvement

PART SEVEN
Shackling the Workforce

PART EIGHT
A New Health Service

Illustrations

Acknowledgements

Many friends and medical colleagues helped me to compile this book, and I am particularly grateful to Dr Fabrizio Casale who gave me access to the Colchester Medical Society's archives.

If I acknowledged everyone who helped, I might run the risk of omitting those who should have been listed, but there are also those who might be embarrassed by being mentioned, because it would appear that they did not wish to be implicated in my interpretation of the state of the NHS and its future rebirth. Therefore I will not acknowledge their contributions, although I am most grateful for those who did help!

None of my contributors were responsible for the narrative, or the way in which I have presented the facts.

Dr Nigel Brayley, who is alas no longer with us, kindly provided illustration 13.

Abbreviations

Preface

In 1948 Nye Heddwyn Selwynne was born. He was the only child of his working class parents, who had tried hard to conceive this cherished baby. Despite the gestation being protracted and the labour complicated and prolonged, the baby was the apple of his parents' eyes. However infancy is a hazardous time in a child's development and his parents fell foul of social services, which decided to take away the child and foster him with a cabal of capitalist cronies.

This should not have been an insurmountable problem, because the child was due to inherit a substantial legacy from the charitable works given over many hundreds of years by well-wishers, but his greedy guardians had other ideas.

After thirteen years of neglect, social services decided that Nye's guardians, Winston, Harold, Alec and Anthony, had failed to bring up the young child according to their rules, and decided to hand back this neglected teenager to some distant working class relatives. However Nye's new guardians were ill prepared for the task, and after seven years of fumbling about, social services handed Nye's future development to Edward and his bossy sister, Margaret.

By this time much of Nye's legacy had been frittered away, and even when a new regime under Tony, the pseudo-socialist, was given the opportunity to make good forty years of neglect, what remained of the family silver was merely given away.

Nye's expectation of life looked poor. He had aged prematurely. None of his guardians had immunised him against the worst diseases of our time, and left with Andrew the antichrist, and Boris the bumbler, all hope of survival seemed to have been lost.

The next chapter of this allegory has not yet been written, but at the present time it looks as though this will in fact be the last chapter.

For anyone, myself included, to claim that in a few hundred pages they could identify the reasons why our National Health Service (NHS) has not been a brilliant success story, and then provide a comprehensive solution to its current problems, is living in cloud-cuckoo-land. However, that should not persuade those of us with the stomach for swallowing bitter criticism, for not attempting to identify the various stumbling blocks which have contributed to the current state of healthcare in the UK.

This is a narrative and not a scientific paper. It is a personal appraisal of healthcare derived from my own experience both as a receiver and a deliverer of medical care. This is not a comprehensive list of all the successes and failures that have shrouded healthcare in the UK, but many of the issues which I have raised in the narrative have been confirmed by colleagues from other parts of the NHS.

Some readers might be annoyed by the way in which I have cobbled together the information in this narrative. I have done this on purpose, in order to encourage those who want to do something about this appalling situation, to make notes as they go along.

In this account I might be considered to be just a Mischievous Arbitrary Fall Guy (MAFG), but someone needs to spell it out.

If the reader wants more details of how the NHS has been emasculated in other parts of the country, there are two excellent publications which give chapter and verse.

1. The Plot against the NHS. Colin Leys & Stewart Player 2011. Merlin Press.

They predicted what would happen if the Health and Social Health (HSC) Act became law.

2. NHS FOR SALE; Myths, Lies & Deception. Jacky Davis, John Lister, David Wrigley 2015. Merlin Press.

They confirmed the predictions of Leys & Player once the legislation became the law, but with even worse consequences.

I started to compile this tome before the Coronavirus pandemic became our preoccupation, and whilst we have always seen the patient as the focus of our attention, we have paid little attention to the welfare of those who play a part in delivering the service. I am not just referring to the doctors and nurses, but everyone from the domestic staff to the junior managers. Maybe I should include all managers and the hospital board, but people who crack the whip, including all politicians, are those who have our blood on their hands.

The other consequence, of our inability to cope with the pandemic, has been an escalation in the number of people, <u>including myself</u>, waiting for hospital appointments, investigations and treatment. The actual numbers are cloaked in the usual statistical governmental fog, but soon it could exceed 8,000,000, and without changes to hospital infrastructure and the working practices of staff, this problem will never be surmounted. Furthermore, this recent paralysis of the NHS has been compounded by the absence of thousands of doctors, and nurses who, irrespective of the presence or absence of symptoms, are self-isolating, often unnecessarily, because of a positive Covid Test, when neither a Lateral Flow nor a PCR test can accurately distinguish between someone actively replicating and disseminating the virus, and someone whose respiratory passages are temporarily contaminated, and not able to spread the disease.
What we really need is a Covid Breathalyser!

In 1948, Britain flirted with a universal scheme of healthcare, but many of the potential participants, especially the Consultants, did not become fully signed up members. Had these doubters boarded the NHS ship as it was boldly launched into the turbulent waters of the ocean of disease, everything might have panned out differently, but within just three years that ship, which had shown so much promise of a fairer society, began to founder, and despite numerous attempts to relaunch it, every rebranding exercise has failed to address the real problems.

Now, seventy four years later, we can see how we currently have a service which has lacked the appropriate level of year on year investment, and has accumulated a massive programme of unfulfilled backlog maintenance.

This is still a complex problem, but by dissecting it limb by limb and organ by organ, perhaps we might succeed in exposing the root causes and explain why we are where we are.

Socialism doesn't sit well in countries whose economies are based on capitalism. Caring for the sick, challenges the boundaries between charity and commerce. London is the second largest money-lending capital in the world, and revenue from the London Stock Market fuels our economy. What little attention capitalists pay to social issues, is done almost grudgingly or because their consciences are pricked.

The birth of the British NHS only came about as a result of the election of a Labour government which had a massive majority in the Houses of Parliament.

Buoyed up by this show of public popularity the new administration thought that they had been given *carte blanche* to deliver their programme to nationalise key industries and set up a nationalised system of healthcare.

Radical changes to the way in which we live require a certain degree of continuity from the people at the top table, so that any glitches in the new systems can be ironed out, but would the electorate give the new government the necessary time to deliver that prize? The British people had just endured six years of death, misery and hardship.

What they wanted in 1945 wasn't more of the same!

What they needed was some TLC, and the socialist government promised to do just that, even though the Treasury had been bankrupted by the previous armed conflict.

Then after only six years of socialist TLC, the electorate was impatient for improvement to their own standards of living, and beguiled by the forked tongues of the Conservative party, which invited them to get back onto the capitalist bandwagon, the people changed horses.

Those good intentions of the Labour Party had neither factored in the time it would take to establish these nationalised organisations, nor the fickle nature of the electorate, but most importantly of all:

Parliament has the authority to denationalise nationalised organisations, and it only takes a parliamentary majority vote to destroy the good intentions of everyone who might have striven to provide our National Health Service.

The six years from 1945-1951 were not long enough to bring about the promised social reform, and during that period of socialism the naysayers had time to develop their plans to derail that socialist dream. Additionally, as people in the post-war era began to accumulate wealth, they became less enamoured with the idea of sharing that wealth with others.

That temporary socialist revolution was over!

It may not have been immediately apparent that the NHS was in the sights of the Conservative Party, but with the public having grown appreciative of free healthcare, the capitalists had to be very careful not to alienate the electorate on whom they depended for their future domination of the political scene.

So any changes the Tories planned to make to the NHS had to be almost undetectable to the man in the street.

Whilst it is easy to blame the Conservative party for the eventual and inevitable deregulation of national healthcare, one must not ignore the passive role played by the medical profession.

The key to the success of the NHS was with the doctors who provided the service but, having put personal gain ahead of the duty of care, they lost the moral high ground and sold their souls and the future of their profession to the devil.

The long term plan of the capitalist politicians was to slowly and methodically extract the teeth from the medical profession. Parliament then had this toothless creature over a barrel.

The doctors remained ambivalent.

They just saw a return to the *status quo* that had been the forerunner to the NHS, but they were misguided.

The accelerating reforms which gathered pace in the 1990s released a score of healthcare related companies gagging at the prospect of getting their noses in the trough and gobbling up any NHS scraps on offer, only to recycle them as pig-shit – a commodity unlikely to fertilise meaningful improvements in healthcare delivery to patients for many decades!

In order to achieve a new nirvana, more sticking plaster will not work. The current legislation will have to be scrapped, and a completely new formula developed.

It will be painful, but without it we will just go muddling aimlessly down the plughole.

Naturally I have selected those parts of this saga which I feel most passionately about.

I have illustrated the way in which the NHS faltered by reference to my own experience as a doctor and patient, and have taken the fate of the hospitals in NE Essex as an example of how the NHS was short-changed, although Colchester was not alone in this situation.

Surprisingly, Colchester's Hospital has survived Special Measures and a takeover by Ipswich Hospital, and despite its campus being littered with Lego, it has acquired some state of the art facilities which seem to have been at the expense of its saviour – Ipswich Hospital. The latest plan is to build a new Orthopaedic Centre on what is currently a hospital car park.

I wonder if Ipswich's catchment population had any say!

As for the London hospitals which bit the bullet, the reader can consult, '**The Lost Hospitals of London**', to see how those closures panned out.

It is up to the reader to decide whether I have been fairly or unfairly biased in my approach.

The last chapter looks at how healthcare in the UK could be revitalised. These are my views and I expect most readers will see this as controversial, especially because in my opinion nothing of any consequence will happen unless the Medical Profession takes the lead, and to do that they will have to accept the culpability of their medical predecessors in aiding and abetting the dismantling of socialist healthcare.

I had hoped to get some help from my former General Practitioner (GP) colleagues, but when I told them that I was writing a book about the NHS, most of them disappeared into the woodwork!

For anyone wishing to discover the complicated way in which GPs are remunerated, they should refer to:

https://www.gov.uk/government/publications/nhs-primary-medical-services-directions-2013

Abbreviations are a bit of a nightmare for those who might come across them for the first time.

Doctors have a long list of such abbreviations, which would mean nothing to anyone outside the medical profession.

When I became a member of the local management committee structure, the abbreviations which the managers used in their communications were difficult to grasp and required an attached list for the purpose of explanation.

For those reasons I have included a list of some but not all of the abbreviations used, and indexed some of the places where they occur in the text. Most of them are in common usage, but others have been invented by me.

When the dust from our present calamitous situation has settled, let us not allow our medical practitioners and nurses to lose sight of their own personal humanitarian vocations, and before we decide where we should be going, we should first discover where we have come from.

Mark Aitken

Leavenheath
March 2022

PART I

Medical Dinosaurs

1

Mediaeval Medicine in England

Practising as a doctor of medicine in mediaeval Britain was a difficult balancing act between success and survival.

Being a patient was probably rather worse!

In the middle ages the non-surgical management of medical conditions was conducted by an odd amalgam of people.

There were the physicians, who had had a classical education and been made aware of macroscopic human anatomy, but with little understanding of how the body functioned.

Then there were various groups of unqualified pretenders, from the village wise woman to the apothecary. They drew the line at surgical intervention, which was left in the hands of the barber-surgeons.

The licensing of this disparate group of 'health' providers started in 1511 when Parliament approved a statute which placed the responsibility for regulation with the bishops.

The bishops were thought to be better qualified to judge between good and evil, and generally saw 'doctors' as people interfering with God's will, after all, if you were destined to live or die then that had been preordained by God and interference by these shady 'medical' characters should be restrained.

The casting out of devils was the duty of the Church.

The real purpose of the 1511 statute was to eliminate 'unqualified' practitioners, and to that end it provided a financial reward for those who reported anyone who lacked the appropriate level of medical education.

The church was never shy of making a few bob!

3

The proper regulation of the medical profession in England didn't start until 1518, when a group of London physicians, led by Thomas Linacre, petitioned King Henry VIII to grant them a charter to control those who were permitted to practice the art of medicine in London. Accordingly they only licenced those, like themselves, who held an Oxbridge medical degree.

The church had been upstaged!

Perhaps we should ask ourselves the question as to why Thomas Linacre and his colleagues started this particular ball rolling.

Was it to safeguard their own livelihood, or to protect the people of London from charlatans?

Was this a charitable act or a commercial wheeze?

It depends on whether we think the best or the worst of our fellow humans.

Maybe it was a bit of both, with some leaning more obviously towards charity and others leaning in the other direction.

In 1523 an Act of Parliament extended the powers of this London based cabal to the whole of England.

In effect these were like fishing licences, which restricted those entitled to fish in their particular pond!

Today there is still that same dichotomy – the schizophrenic dual personality of those who deliver healthcare.

It is all about motivation, and mankind's motivation is driven by his quest to control the environment in which he works and lives.

In the sixteenth century there was very little science in the art of medical practice, so the possession of an Oxbridge medical degree was unlikely to have offered much protection to the public.

At that time physicians played no part in carrying out surgical procedures which had remained the remit of the Guild of Barber Surgeons since the 14th century, and their operations were

4

considered to be 'barbaric' by the snooty physicians – and probably rightly so!

It wasn't until 1745 that the surgeons broke away from the barbers to form the Company of Surgeons, which later became the Royal College of Surgeons (RCS).

In Scotland a rather different approach had been adopted.

In Glasgow, Peter Lowe received a royal charter from King James VI in 1599 to form the Glasgow Faculty of Physicians, Surgeons and Dentists, and in 1909 this became the Royal Faculty of Physicians and Surgeons of Glasgow (RFPSG).

In Edinburgh a royal charter was granted in 1681 for Sir Robert Sibbald to form a college of physicians which then became the Royal College of Physicians of Edinburgh (RCPE).

In 1505 surgery followed a similar pattern to that adopted in London where the Barber Surgeons had become a craft guild, and much later acquired the title of the Royal College of Surgeons of Edinburgh (RCSE).

All the Scottish medical colleges were responsible for the regulation and education of those aspiring to become physicians, surgeons or dentists.

However, in spite of these learned bodies leading the way, there was the need for something a bit more all-inclusive.

2

Victorian and Edwardian Britain

In 1832, Sir Charles Hastings convened a meeting in the Board Room of Worcester Infirmary, and in the presence of fifty doctors, proposed the founding of the *Provincial Medical and Surgical Association* (PMSA) ostensibly for the sharing of scientific knowledge between doctors.

Ten years after this initial meeting the association's membership had grown to 1350 and it had begun to publish a weekly journal, '*The Provincial Medical and Surgical Journal*', known from 1857 onwards as the *British Medical Journal* or BMJ.

The association's membership grew rapidly and in 1853 the PMSA extended its membership to London doctors and became the *British Medical Association* or BMA in 1856.

Although not initially formed with the aim of initiating medical reform, the Association's *Parliamentary Bills Committee*, played a key role in the drafting and passing of the Medical Act of 1858, and took a leading role in influencing legislation on Public Health. The Medical Act established *The General Council of Medical Education and Registration of the United Kingdom*, which later became known as the *General Medical Council* (GMC).

This body declared that doctors licensed by them would enable patients who sought medical advice to distinguish between qualified and unqualified practitioners.

In effect the GMC became the new professional regulator, but would the GMC carry the can if they erroneously licenced an unqualified doctor?

There was an instance in Clacton where the GMC had licenced a person whose only previous medical experience had been that of a medical student! He had passed no medical examination! It was only after several years, when the local GPs became suspicious of his medical expertise, that the error was uncovered. Is the GMC in reality just a CMG – Crafty Money Grubber?

With the GMC taking over licencing, the medical colleges needed to find a new source of income, and this was fulfilled by the provision of postgraduate education and the awarding of postgraduate qualifications. These degrees, such as the MRCP and FRCS, then became the necessary credentials for obtaining Consultant positions, and saw the beginning of the medical nonsense of *multiple diplomatosis*.

By 1900 there were all sorts of medical professional bodies, from the surgeons and dentists to the psychiatrists, all vying to control and feed off this medical arena.

Close on the coattails of these burgeoning sources of medical assistance came the money chandlers, selling health insurance policies to anyone gullible enough not to realise that no matter how much you pay up front, these vagabonds are in it not to safeguard your health, but to make a nice little profit from the almost invisible small print which beguiles those who gamble with chance!

From the middle of the nineteenth century onwards, with the application of medical gases, such as diethyl ether (ether), nitrous oxide and chloroform, to produce general anaesthesia during surgery, the scope of surgical practice expanded rapidly.

The surgeon no longer had to race through a procedure with only opium and alcohol to deaden the pain being inflicted upon the patient.

Now they could take their time and use their knowledge of human anatomy and their manual dexterity to perform meticulous operations which had previously only been pipe dreams.

For the physician, the discovery and isolation of pathogenic bacteria; the application of haematology and chemical

8

pathology to blood testing; and the use of imaging with x-rays; all contributed to a better understanding of disease and now there was a bit more than intuitive guesswork to making a correct or incorrect diagnosis!

With the prospect of recovery from medical conditions, instead of certain death or hoping for a miraculous outcome, more and more people availed themselves of medical assistance, irrespective of whether or not they were covered by insurance. However medical fees soared, and with that there was a realisation, that when medical or surgical intervention did not live up to a patient's expectations, then the disgruntled patient could sue for malpractice.

There followed a corresponding explosion of patients suing for damages, so that by the 1880s it became essential for medical practitioners to insure themselves against litigation from aggrieved patients. However, the BMA, to which many doctors belonged, was not permitted under its constitution to undertake individual medical defence.

In 1885, a group of solicitors signed a memorandum that established the aims and objectives of their newly registered company, the *Medical Defence Union* (MDU). They backed up their action by alluding to the outrage in the medical community over the case of a Dr David Bradley who had been wrongly convicted of a charge of assaulting a woman in his surgery.

Dr Bradley spent eight months in prison before receiving a full pardon.

The annual subscription cost MDU members 10 shillings.

This denouement was followed in 1892 by the establishment of the (*London and Counties) Medical Protection Society* (MPS), and within two years it had more than 1,000 members.

The medical insurance industry had become a highly competitive and profitable business, but the politicians also wanted a slice of the cake.

The 1911 National Insurance Act was the brainchild of the Liberal Party's Chancellor of the Exchequer, David Lloyd George, who adapted the German system which had been introduced in 1884 by the German Chancellor, Otto von Bismarck.

This Liberal legislation gave the British working classes the first state sponsored contributory system of insurance against illness and unemployment, but it only applied to wage earners, i.e. about 70% of the work force, and their families.

This ushered in the foundations of the modern welfare state.

The medical profession as a whole opposed this intrusion of government into territory which they considered to be sacrosanct, and the majority of Conservative MPs voted against this Bill. However, they would bide their time and wait for the appropriate opportunity to facilitate the unravelling of this misplaced act of politicised charity.

Naturally working people welcomed this denouement.

Those who earned under £160 a year had to pay 4 pence a week to the scheme; the employer paid 3 pence, and general taxation contributed 2 pence.

This entitled workers and their families to free consultation and treatment by a 'panel doctor' for various medical conditions including tuberculosis.

In due course maternity benefits were included.

Furthermore, workers could take sick leave and be paid 10 shillings a week for the first 13 weeks, and 5 shillings a week for the next 13 weeks.

The employers were not too pleased, because it burdened them with the bureaucracy and the cost of collecting and then transferring the funds.

At the beginning these contributions were sent to the employees' relevant Union or Friendly Society, for them to administer as needs arose.

The insurance companies were quick to seize this opportunity and set up their own, 'government approved' bodies to handle these funds, but in due course the government took charge of this free for all and, in the name of the National Insurance Fund, started to collect and administer the benefits, whilst at the same time reducing the tax payers' contributions!

There was a key assumption pertaining to this Act – namely that the unemployment rate would not exceed 4.6%.
At the time the Act was passed, unemployment was only 3%, and the fund was expected to build up a substantial surplus, but to many this smelled of the government collecting money for old rope!

In the meantime, the 30% of the population, who were not covered by this scheme, had to make their own arrangements in regard to medical and unemployment insurance, and resented the fact they were also subsidising the National Insurance Fund through general taxation.

3

The Polarisation of Society

In the increasingly protectionist attitude towards ill-health, there was a need to protect the upper echelons of society from the poor and the contagion of mental, physical and infectious diseases, not forgetting the criminal fraternity.

Prisons were built for those criminals who could not be hanged or sent to Australia. The poor could be forcibly contained in the Work House. The mentally reprehensible could be hidden away in Lunatic Asylums and those with contagious diseases could be herded together in Fever Hospitals.

These measures made communities more pleasant to live in, but not more humane.

The Fever Hospitals provided sensible Public Health measures in order to contain and limit the spread of communicable diseases. The spectre of the plagues and epidemics of previous times haunted those given the responsibility for protecting the health of the public.

Every English borough had to find the financial resources to maintain this service, and the local taxpayer footed the bill.

Mental health was another deeply divisive area of healthcare and once again the local community grudgingly footed the bill, although they valued the removal of 'mad' people from their neighbourhoods. Unfortunately the definition of madness was open to abuse so that, for example, an unmarried mother could be sent to a Lunatic Asylum, and in one case a girl who, having allegedly attempted to drown herself in a basin of water, was confined to a mental subnormality asylum for decades despite having an Intelligence Quotient (IQ) of 120!

There was also the ability of sane members of the community to seek asylum in these institutions.

Most towns also had a charitable hospital or infirmary.

These had been founded long before medical practice had much to offer the sick. The building of these infirmaries and their maintenance and administration relied wholly upon charitable donations. Initially the money came from bequests, but in due course it became necessary to nominate days in the year when donations were collected in the streets from passers-by.

In Gloucester a charity pageant to pay off the debts of the local infirmary raised £10,800 – mostly in the form of large donations from the great and the good.

In Glasgow £10,300 was collected during a Saturday afternoon, but that included six tons in pennies, bawbees (halfpennies) and farthings donated by the indigent poor!

In 1907 a special fund was set up by the management committee of Colchester's Essex County Hospital (ECH) so that children could be nursed in accommodation separated from adults.

Local children were encouraged to donate enough to buy a brick!

Within just one year, not only had the capital been raised but the children's ward had been built and opened by H.R.H. Princess Louise!

When the charitable and caring nature of mankind is appropriately motivated, almost anything seemed to be possible, but healthcare in general, before the NHS, was slow to adopt best practice.

In 1946, when I was eight years old, almost 40 years after ECH had built their Paediatric Ward, I was admitted to the male surgical ward of the Royal Naval Hospital in Chatham.

There was no Paediatric Ward.

Children < 5 years of age were admitted to the female wards.

Children >5 years of age were placed in a line of beds down the centre of the adult wards.

There were no screens.

Night-time ushered in the worst nightmare, when a deathly white victim of the latest surgical procedure was wheeled down the ward on a trolley spattered with blood, and then humped unceremoniously onto a neighbouring bed.

Days later the same person was wheeled out in a metal box.

Then a new incumbent, admitted in a similar way, took his place.

Four weeks spent in that environment, followed by abandonment in a children's convalescent home deep in the Kent countryside for the best part of five months, was an experience which I will never forget.

Why did it take so long for the medical profession to realise that children should be separated from adults in the hospital environment?

4

The Need for Change

Right up until the 1940s, medical and surgical practice was run either by local voluntary/charitable hospitals, local authority funded institutions or private medical practices and hospitals.

People in need of medical care could either go to a local GP, or present themselves to the nearest hospital Casualty department.

In both cases this would involve a fee which was payable at the point of access, although the GP might waive the fee for the most indigent patients, and the hospital Almoner might provide the funds for the poorest and most needy.

Clearly charity was available, but the patient really needed to deserve it!

The part played by the voluntary/charitable hospital's in the local community can best be illustrated by reference to the role of the ECH in Colchester, and expertly explained in John Penfold's book, 'The History of the Essex County Hospital, Colchester'.

This hospital was founded in 1820 for the care of the sick indigent poor of the town and its environs. It was supported by charitable donations, legacies and fund raising initiatives.

By the 1920s the hospital had thrown off its image as a place where the sick might more likely than not die of their ailments, to a hive of entrepreneurial endeavour, but the hospital was still largely speaking supported by charity.

Nonetheless inpatients were charged £1 per week, and outpatients one shilling per visit, if they could afford to pay.

However a local insurance scheme was in operation at that time whereby, for the regular payment of twopence per week, inpatient charges would be waived.

The hospital was run by a group of local honorary GPs, who decided which patients should be seen as outpatients and which patients were worthy of admission.

A record of the annual salaries of staff at the end of the nineteenth century was recorded in Dr Penfold's book as follows:

Salaried Physician	£200
House Surgeon/Apothecary	£100
Matron	£60
Nurse (average)	£24
Dispenser	£65
Porter	£27
Cook	£24
Housemaid	£12
Hospital Secretary	£140
Kitchen Maid	£10
Ward Maid	£9

All the other qualified medical practitioners gave their services without receiving a penny. They derived their income solely from their individual general practices.

All the surgical procedures were performed free of charge by these GPs, except that with the establishment of some private accommodation as early as 1900, and a bespoke private ward in 1927 (with a complement of twelve cubicles), the hospital was able to obtain an additional source of income to offset its charitable work, and the GPs were able to charge those patients for services rendered.

The hospital's income from private patients and the local insurance scheme contributed over 50% to the cost of running the hospital.

The real change in the way in which surgery was performed did not happen until Dr Ronnie Reid arrived in Colchester.

Although he was only 23 years of age, he had already obtained the degree of Master of Surgery (MS), and was a FRCS.

In order to practise his surgical skills at the hospital, he had to be a local GP, so he went into practice with Drs Perceval, Reddington and Fripp. However, within three years he gave up general practice and just worked at the ECH, where his services to the general public were free, but he earned his living by operating on private patients, who understandably flocked to see him.

This *volte face* got up the noses of the local GPs, whose surgical abilities were way below those of this highly qualified surgeon.

There was also the stigma of having a private ward in an essentially charitable hospital, and the need to conceal its existence from general scrutiny.

This private facility had been added to the floor above the newly constructed outpatient department, and thus slipped in under the radar. This obfuscation was sealed by naming the new ward 'Jefferson Ward', in honour of one of the hospital's founding fathers, who might well have turned in his grave at this blatant deceit!

At no time did the hospital take on a maternity service, except where complicated obstetric situations arose, but the hospital environment was not ideal for these women.

In 1932 a large private house, just under a mile from the hospital, was opened as Colchester's Maternity Home.

Over the ensuing years it grew rapidly in size, and the local GPs, who oversaw the management of these pregnant women, preferred the new arrangements and its relative freedom from the hassle and potential source of infection, which compromised the management of pregnancies which had already become complicated.

Charitable contributions in time and effort came from many sources and in particular the development of the Colchester blood transfusion service by Mr Alec Blaxill, a partner of the local builders merchants. He had no medical or relevant scientific qualifications, but had enthusiasm in spades!

In a short space of time he had recruited a panel of about 2,000 potential donors, who were individually brought by him, day or night, to the hospital or maternity home as and when blood was required in an emergency!

Furthermore, after such emergencies had been resuscitated, Mr Blaxill would send a card to the donor or donors, informing them of the recipients state of recovery.

In the ten years before the NHS was founded, ECH had changed from a place where GPs treated and operated upon their patients, to a hospital with *bona fide* career Consultants without either foot in the general practice milieu. The scope of treatments available for patients increased without any significant change in mortality, but this did increase the cost of running the hospital, despite the new Consultants still giving their services to the local population free of charge, unless they were private patients.

By the end of the Second World War (WWII), the state of health provision in the UK was on its knees.

Despite most people having some sort of private or government sponsored medical insurance, the hospitals were in desperate need of financial investment.

To its credit, ECH had balanced its books as a result of disposing of all its property and assets. However, that left it vulnerable, and without some sort of national takeover, it would fail.

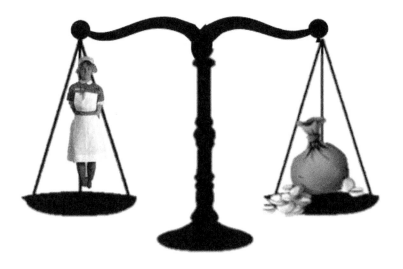

Balance of Healthcare in Britain before WWII

PART II

A Social Revolution

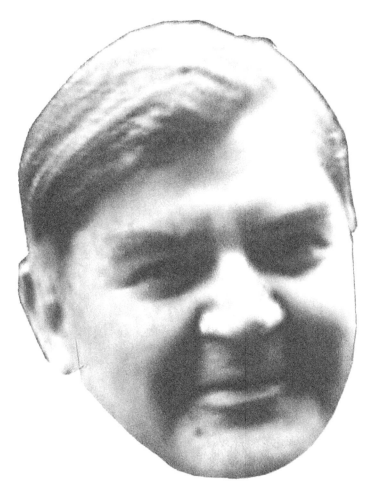

Hello Aneurin Bevan (Nye)

5

The New Beginning

Britain may have played an important role in defeating Nazi Germany, but she was on her knees and heavily in debt to the USA for the military assistance we had received, but not yet paid for, prior to the USA deciding to throw their hat into the ring.

The people of Britain were fed up with austerity and rationing. They wanted a better quality of life without the Haves taking all the cake from the Have-Nots.

The charitable hospitals had run out of money, and their erstwhile capitalist benefactors did not or could not afford to volunteer to step into the breech.

From 1935-1945 the Conservatives had a parliamentary majority of 171 seats. During the coalition government from 1940-1945 the Minister of Health (Sir Henry Urmston Willink) drew up a white paper on a possible comprehensive free healthcare system 'A National Health Service', which proposed the creation of such a service, but without including the nationalisation of hospitals. He consulted widely including members of the Labour Party and in particular Nye Bevan.

He also noted the sterling work carried out by the social reformer, Sir William Beveridge, whose report, published in 1942, outlined the need to address the five evils of the time namely: poverty, ignorance, squalor, idleness and disease.

At that time Beveridge only briefly (1944-45) became an MP (as a result of a by-election).

It is uncertain whether Nye Bevan held any official post in the Department of Health (DoH), but news of the formulation of this white paper was no secret, and it encouraged the lobbying of certain interested parties from Wales.

Henry Richard Jones, a leading figure in the Medical Aid Societies of South Wales, fearing that a bill would be passed with the concerns of the Welsh not being considered, contacted Bevan requesting an audience with the Minister. However, Bevan wasn't in a position to complicate the already tense situation, and tried to pacify the Welsh, after all, he had been a leading light in the Tredegar Medical Aid Society, which had provided medical services to miners and workers through the collection of small weekly contributions.

Bevan knew that, with a few modifications, the Welsh system could be adapted to fit the whole of the British population, but he also knew, when Sir Henry Willink's White Paper was published in 1944, that the massive Conservative majority in Parliament was likely to kill it ever coming into law.

All Bevan needed to do was to bide his time and wait for the Labour Party to be at the helm of British politics.

It should have been no surprise to an outsider that in the 1945 General Election the Labour Party under Clement Atlee went on to win a 494/640 landslide victory, giving them a majority of 146 in Parliament.

With that sort of majority they probably felt that they could move heaven and earth!

The Tory Party – the great advocates of capitalism – couldn't believe what had happened.

Was it not the Conservative imperialist politicians who had taken us into two catastrophic, although eventually victorious, world wars?

Was Winston Churchill not an iconic figure in war, and now deserved recognition in peace?

Where was our gratitude for the benevolence of his followers?

However, the Labour Party had earned a mandate through the ballot box to deliver a fairer more equitable society!

Key aspects of commerce would be nationalised, and a health service for all, irrespective of means, would be established. This was the setting for the NHS.

In every takeover deal there is a lot of small print to be made legally watertight.

1. Taking ownership of the land, the buildings and their contents.
2. Partially reimbursing the hospitals' creditors.
3. Renewing contracts with suppliers.
4. Removing all the parasites which had been feeding off healthcare.
5. Negotiating new employment contracts with staff.

Many of the Charity/Voluntary Hospitals were not fit for purpose, and could be rebuilt or relocated more appropriately. However, although Nye Bevan was the Minister of Health, he was also the Minister for Housing, and that gave him the additional opportunity to use the land, acquired under the NHS Act, for the construction of desperately needed social housing. Naturally the construction industry, which was in private hands, welcomed this increase in business activity. The Government had some say in the quality of housing to be built, but could not control the profits made by the builders, who must have thought they had won a lottery.

The attitude of the medical profession towards the proposed NHS was negative, or at best ambivalent. One might have expected the doctors to have embraced the principles of universal healthcare, but at the top of the profession were three medical dinosaurs, which had personal axes to grind, and points to be scored over each other.

1. Charles Hill – secretary of the BMA.
2. Charles Wilson – president of the RCP.
3. Thomas Horder – private physician to the monarchy and many important politicians.

Charles Hill represented the majority of family doctors, and they were worried about the possibility of becoming salaried employees of the state, and little more than civil servants, who had to bow to every whim and fancy of the non-medical political elite.

Thomas Horder sided with Charles Hill, and had the support of a substantial number of hospital Consultants, who strongly opposed the creation of a free Public Health service and the possibility of losing both kudos and earnings from Private Practice. Horder also hoped that, with so many Consultants backing him, he would be elected as the next President of the RCP – something he had been trying to achieve for the last decade.

Charles Wilson, who had been and still was the personal physician to Winston Churchill, knew a bit or two about manipulating others, and had already earned the nickname 'Corkscrew Charlie'!

The three protagonists fought over the spoils, but it was Charles Wilson who had Bevan's ear, and it was he who fashioned the new contract between the government and the medical profession.

Once the infighting was over, it was clear to anyone who cared to look at the details, that the medical profession could be bought, in Bevan's own words, 'filling their mouths with gold'!
It was rather like the fairy tale about the man who had lost his shadow, or Faust's pact with the Devil.

6

The Day of Reckoning

The launch of the NHS on 5th July 1948 was viewed by the electorate with a mixture of misgiving and elation.

Wealthier citizens, who already had some form of health insurance, viewed this denouement as a levelling down of the playing field, because they saw themselves having to share these new amenities with the great unwashed.

The poorer members of the community saw this beacon of light as a sorely needed measure of social justice, and a levelling up of the playing field.

Either way, launching the NHS in the summer, when the pressure on the health service was likely to be low, was a wise move, because it gave the population time to go through the formalities of registering with a family practitioner before the winter surge in demand dominated the attention of those charged with delivering healthcare.

The forerunner for this launch date had been a nationwide advertising campaign which began in February 1948.

It described in detail how people should go about registering with a GP, what services would be available to them, how to get dental treatment, sight and hearing tests, and everything else that might impinge on their state of wellbeing.

It was interesting to note that even as the NHS was born, Bevan stated that it might be necessary in the future to expect patients to make a financial contribution towards their care.

In fact it took just three years before false teeth and spectacles fell into this category.

During July 1948 GPs gritted their teeth and waited for an inrush of demand, but during the first few weeks it was all about filing the forms which had been completed by people wishing to register, and agreeing to add them to their list.

This was merely an exercise in administration.

Some doctors cancelled or postponed their summer holidays in order not to miss the boat while other practices were taking 'passengers on board'.

The charity hospitals, which were already pretty well insolvent, waited anxiously to see if their services would be axed or transferred elsewhere.

Those hospitals which were just about solvent were allowed to retain any remaining endowments, but the endowments of struggling hospitals were confiscated by the Treasury.

The teaching hospitals had special arrangements.

In England, these hospitals were allowed to keep their endowments and their property portfolios

In Scotland, endowments were pooled to form the Scottish Hospitals Endowments Research Trust (SHERT), and would in future be used to support medical research projects in Scotland.

This complemented the activities of the Medical Research Council (MRC) in England, which had been set up in principle if not in name before 1914. Efforts were made in subsequent years to ensure that the MRC was separate from government and would make decisions about funding research projects irrespective of the colour of the government in power.

Sadly the medical profession in general did not demand a similar stance in regard to the way in which the government allocated NHS funds for the maintenance and enhancement of the healthcare environment, but perhaps it was the spectre of a conflict of interest which chased this ghost into the shadows.

Patients living near a teaching hospital could avail themselves of treatment there, just as they had done before 1948, but in that situation they were initially likely to be seen by a medical student.

7

First Impressions

It is easy to imagine that everything that happened after July 1948 was attributable to the new NHS, but the provision of healthcare didn't stand still while the outcome of the negotiations between the Government and the Profession were grinding on.

The capital funding of new technologies and replacement of old equipment had been a particular headache for the voluntary hospitals. It usually meant the launching of fresh appeals for the local community to dig deep into their pockets.

These were donations, not loans.

In that regard, the installation of a radiotherapy department would be hard to justify.

Although radiotherapy had been around for almost fifty years, it was still a relatively novel treatment for cancer, and was used predominantly to mop up the remnants of cancerous tissue that the surgeons had been unable to remove. It was also used to treat cancers of the skin, and benign conditions such as cavernous haemangiomas and ankylosing spondylitis.

Radiotherapy had become part of the treatment profile offered by the Teaching Hospitals, but with the exception of the inhabitants of London, patients had to travel long distances in order to avail themselves of this treatment modality. In this regard the Radiotherapy Department of the London Hospital served a small part of the city, and also the whole of Essex. Their department risked being overwhelmed by the sheer work load, and thereby unable to develop more sophisticated ways of enhancing the modality's capability.

At that time, Dr Frank Ellis, the director of the Radiotherapy Department, began to explore the possibility of organising the follow-up of his patients from Essex closer to their homes, and to that end started follow-up clinics in Romford and Colchester.

In 1947, with the prospect of the proposed NHS being able to fund satellite Radiotherapy Departments, Dr Ellis suggested that Dr Rhys Lewis, his Senior Registrar, might take over the Colchester follow-up clinic on his behalf, with a view to the ultimate installation of an orthovoltage machine for Dr Rhys Lewis to treat superficially located neoplasms.

All that was needed to seal the deal was for the NHS to become law, and an appropriate bid for capital funding to be approved by the NE Thames Metropolitan Region Hospital Board (NETMRB).

This plan resonated with the Labour Government's ethos of decentralizing services and curtailing the enrichment of the major hospitals in London – the capital of capitalism.

This was how Dr Rhys Lewis was appointed as Colchester's Consultant Radiotherapist; how radiotherapy found a niche in Colchester; how this service first turned out to be an asset; and then became a handicap to the future development of healthcare in NE Essex.

The new health service also made it possible to pay those who had previously given their services without enjoying any financial reward. The payment of hospital Consultants, for personal services rendered, had been a sticking point in the negotiations between the Labour Government and the Medical Profession. The fear that Private Practice would dry up as soon as the NHS became law, was the rationale for allowing Consultants, who joined the NHS hospital service, to continue to feed from the private healthcare market.

However, within a short period of time any worries that hospital Consultants might have had, about the new scheme decimating their Private Practice, were quickly assuaged.

In fact, Private Practice boomed regardless.

The NHS act had at a stroke increased hospital Consultant salaries, by paying them for the services which they had previously provided completely freely!

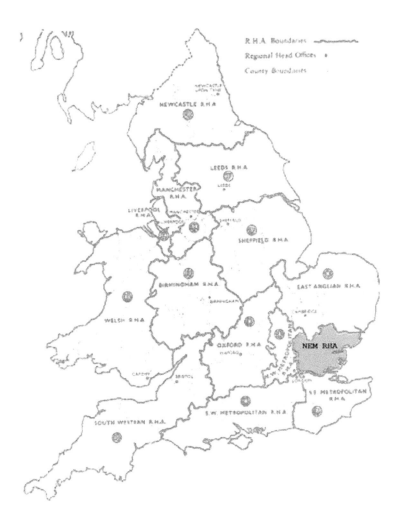

NHS England & Wales Regional Health Authorities

8

Managing the New National Charity

Prior to the NHS takeover of medical practice in the UK, the Charity or Voluntary Hospital had been managed by a committee comprising several local GPs, some local bigwigs and a 'Secretary'.

The Secretary received a salary and effectively implemented the decisions made by the Committee. The other members of the Committee received no financial reward for their services, but might benefit indirectly if they owned a relevant local business which provided goods to the hospital.

The GPs continued to earn their living from providing their services to the paying community.

The Government played no part in this arrangement, although from time to time and during armed conflicts it did provide grants to struggling hospitals.

With the inception of the NHS, two layers of political management were placed above the hospital management committee, namely the Minister of Health and his Ministry, which received their funding from the Treasury, and in England and Wales there were 14 new Regional Boards, such as the NETMRB, which now oversaw the activity of Essex, NE London and a part of Hertfordshire, i.e. a whole bunch of salaried managers to eat up part of the money earmarked for healthcare!

The 14 regions were initially supposed to represent areas with similarly sized populations, but this did not take account of the level of social deprivation nor the inaccessibility of hospital services to people living in rural areas. Furthermore, in the South Western RHA the distance from the most southerly parts of Cornwall to the RHA offices in Bristol was about 180 miles, and that gave the inhabitants of Cornwall the impression that they received less funding than they deserved.

Scotland and Northern Ireland had their own management systems tailored to the needs of their own 'devolved' regions.

The funding of the hospital service had to take its place in the queue of other health related services now under the umbrella of the DoH, and alongside the other government ministries knocking at the doors of the Treasury, such as the Ministries of Defence, Education, Housing, Transport, etc, etc.

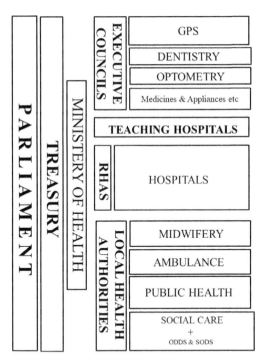

Sharing the Health Budget in England & Wales

It might have made more sense, at the start of this departmental free-for-all, to have ring fenced the budget of the Ministry of

Health (MOH), and fed it through a different source of taxation, such as the National Insurance Scheme, even if by so doing there would need to be new legislation. Furthermore, since Social Care was also funded by local taxation, it would be all too easy to reduce that part of the Health Ministry's responsibility, and dump it at the doors of the County and Borough Councils.

Sleight of hand by politicians was well recognised, but would the Medical Profession shine out from the mire of politics and set an example?

Unfortunately not!

Conflicts of interest were not slow to present themselves to the Medical Profession.

The ability of doctors to enjoy the benefits of providing care to both private and NHS patients required a level of honesty which was over and above that expected of the general public. Although Bevan had wanted to create a strict dividing line between the private and public service offered by doctors, he had to bow to the demands of the profession.

In the 1948 Act there was no clause which would allow a change to this demarcation line.

Thus there was the opportunity for the doctor to accept the fee offered by the patient and claim the going rate from the government, whilst earning a salary from the government for providing that healthcare.

Nobody in the ministry was likely to suss out the deception!

Could the doctor or dentist accept what was offered by the patient as a tip in the same way as the taxi driver?

Should gifts offered by patients at Christmas be declared on one's tax return?

Once this line had been crossed the temptation remained!

Furthermore, the hospital service was not alone in the field of those providing healthcare and ready to exploit this new marketplace.

It was the responsibility of the Executive Councils to manage the needs and greeds of this tranche of healthcare.

41

Prior to 1948, some GPs did their own dispensing and charged patients accordingly. If they continued to provide this service they naturally expected some form of extra funding over and above what they received as a capitation fee for every patient registered at their practice.

Then there were minor surgical procedures which they had previously performed on the premises. If they were to continue providing that local service, then they expected extra remuneration, otherwise they would just refer these patients to the local hospital.

These little enhancements then became the thin end of a wedge which ultimately landed them with having to take on extra top-down politicized functions, straight from the DoH.

Chemist shops, otherwise known as pharmacies, dispensed medicines and appliances prescribed by GPs. Making a profit on what they supplied to NHS patients was to be expected, although not in the spirit of the NHS.

Their 'dispensing fees' required additional legislation, and were hotly contested by the pharmacists own professional bodies.

Dentists occupied a different position in the scheme of things, because patients did not have to register with a dentist, in the same way that they needed to register with a GP. It was up to the dentist to decide into which category a patient seeking treatment should fall, i.e. Private or NHS.

Dentists were perhaps the first, amongst those who had been placed under the umbrella of the Executive Council, to enjoy a financial bonanza, particularly in underprivileged areas of the country, where dental caries was rife and edentulous patients abounded.

For these patients a pair of false teeth meant that they would at last be able to enjoy a meal that required a degree of biting, chewing or grinding!

On the other side of this new administrative pathway were the services which had previously been provided by the local county, borough and town councils, and paid for by local taxation.

The grant received from the DoH in order to continue those services was a welcome relief for local taxpayers. It also gave local government the opportunity to enhance and rationalize the services which they provided, but also allowed them to become dependent upon the associated government handouts.

In the fullness of time they would become vassals of national political agendas, which in turn depended upon the colour of the party in power.

Cutting government grants to the communities meant that services might need to be curtailed, particularly when new governments started to limit the level of taxation, which local councils could levy from their communities!

As they say, 'when you sup with the devil, you need to use a very long spoon'!

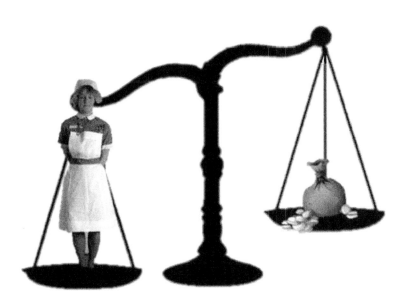

Proposed Balance of Healthcare in 1948

PART III

Working Within the NHS 1962-1975

9

On Becoming Junior Doctors

For those of us who had enrolled as medical students in the 1950s and 1960s, we had little understanding of what healthcare had been like before 1948. In our five or six years in medical school we learned how science had shaped medical practice, and most of us believed that science would lead us into a world where disease became less of a threat to man's way of life.

Our vision was focussed on the way ahead, and how we would achieve our goals. We had little idea of the medically irrelevant factors which had already shaped and would continue to shape the outcome of the NHS, although we had been aware of the bizarre way in which we had originally been selected to train as doctors.

Most Teaching Hospitals had their own preclinical schools, where prospective school leavers were interviewed before being offered a place. After two years, and having passed the preclinical exams, there was automatic acceptance to proceed into the hospital environment without any additional interview.

For those who had obtained exemption from taking the Teaching Hospital's preclinical exam, by virtue of having obtained a degree after spending three years 'reading' a Natural Sciences Tripos or its equivalent at one of Britain's universities, one had to jump the next hurdle into the clinical environment. This involved being selected at interview by one of the Teaching Hospitals.

One might have thought that, after having successfully mastered the medical sciences, such an interview would concentrate on the suitability of the applicant for a life as a doctor, but my experience was rather different.

My first interview was a Guy's Hospital.
The interview committee consisted of the Dean and four other consultants arranged around a table, with me sitting opposite the Dean. The interviewers took turns to ask a selection of seemingly bizarre questions for which I had had no well thought out answers.
When I left the room I saw another of my erstwhile undergraduate contemporaries waiting to be interviewed. He had never impressed me as being the sort of person who would make a good doctor.
When I heard that he had been accepted by Guy's, whereas I had been rejected, I wondered what those interviewers had found so special about his candidacy.
My next interview was at St Bartholomew's Hospital (Barts).
The interview was conducted by Mr Ellison Nash (the Dean) – a Paediatric Consultant Surgeon.
The first and only question was, 'Do you believe in God?'
How does one answer that when one was already questioning the existence of a divine deity?
I fumbled my way through the next minute, and then was entertained by the Dean to a ten minute discourse on Christianity.
While waiting to hear whether I had been accepted by Barts, I toyed with the idea to applying to the Middlesex Hospital or University College Hospital, but wondered if their caricatured names as, the 'Yiddlesex' and the 'JewCH' respectively, might require me to adopt a new religion!

I was accepted by Barts and enjoyed the subsequent training experience. Much later I discovered that the Dean was accepting anyone, provided that they were not accredited Welsh rugby players!
So much for deciding whether or not a prospective student had what it would take to be a good doctor!
At the same time there was an interesting statistic – only 10% of medical students in London were female.
Today that figure is more like 60%.
With a limited number of places for medical students to study, this excluded many potential male school leavers from becoming doctors, because boys usually had somewhat less spectacular A Level grades than girls. Sexual equality in the workplace is all well and good, but how might this impact adversely on the future staffing of the medical workforce? Women have their unique natural quality – the ability to reproduce the species, but this would

48

invariably take them away from their healthcare functions, and leave gaps that would need to be filled if the service had to continue without any blips. Consequently today, many female doctors are employed on a 'part-time' basis, especially in general practice.

With the need for more doctors to cope with the increasing size of the population, especially the elderly, this sex ratio is likely to have an adverse effect on our ability to provide a comprehensive medical workforce!

Once we had qualified, we had to complete two six month hospital appointments, as House Surgeon and House Physician, before becoming fully licenced by the GMC.

It was only then that we could plan the way ahead.

The majority opted for either Hospital Practice or General Practice. A few chose the Laboratory Services or Public Health, whilst the remainder sat on the fence and bided their time.

We were totally blind to the political undercurrent which would bubble up intermittently and slowly erode the nature of healthcare.

For us the schedule of work was arduous.

There was an alternate night duty rota, one weekend in two free, and just two weeks paid annual leave, but the experience was second to none, and for those of us who saw medical practice as a vocation, it was psychologically very rewarding.

The pay was not great but, with the majority of us living on the hospital premises, there was little time in which to spend our salaries. Furthermore, on becoming a Consultant or GP, the financial and social rewards were very enticing.

At this time very few junior doctors were married, but marriage soon began to shape our direction of travel. Family life is complicated if one regularly has to be on duty at night and weekends. Unless one's spouse was fully aware of this disrupting effect and accepted it with good grace, one's choice of future employment became limited.

One might think that with increasing numbers of patients in need of medical attention, there would be every prospect of finding a good practice to join or getting promotion in the hospital environment, but there was one major fly in the ointment which snared the path ahead.

Those who had already obtained Consultant status were loath to share their cake with others. They selfishly ensured that there was a limit to the number of junior doctors who could fill the posts of Senior Registrar, and that number was geared to be sufficient to replace existing Consultants when either they retired or fell by the wayside.

This led to there being a bottleneck in the system at the level of medical or surgical registrar.

Many doctors marooned in this grade, who had achieved the necessary postgraduate qualifications required to fill a Consultant post, grew tired of the impasse and became GPs, thus enhancing the professionalism and scope of General Practice.

The same overqualified doctor might also acquire a hospital appointment as a 'clinical assistant' to a nominated Consultant and act as a sort of supernumerary Senior Registrar.

The enterprising future GP realised that having a few extra qualifications might put them in good stead for the better GP Practice vacancies, and therefore spent some time as Senior House Officers (SHOs) in Obstetrics & Gynaecology (O&G) and/or Paediatrics, thereby obtaining the Diplomas from the Royal College of O&G (DRCOG) or a Diploma of Child Health (DCH).

As the population grew so the number of GPs attached to each practice increased, in order to meet this demand and the variation in patient needs. This was affordable so long as each new patient came with their individually wrapped annual capitation fee, and there were no unnecessary strings attached by government.

Of course the politicians couldn't resist the desire to offer alternative ways to enhance GP salaries, whilst shackling them with a tsunami of bureaucratic paperwork.

This caused the GP to be distracted from the care of patients and towards the comfort of the politicians.

Medicine had lost its focus and its vocation.

In the 1960s, the junior hospital doctor was part of a firm which typically comprised of a Pre-registration House Officer (PRHO), maybe a SHO if you were lucky, and a Registrar. The nominal leader – the Consultant – played a rather 'hands off' role, in so far as one rarely saw the leader except on the two statutory weekly ward rounds.

In my case, as a medical PRHO at a hospital out in the sticks, those ward rounds started, at 8.30 am, and finished about an hour later with me running beside the Consultant's car taking the last instructions through the open car window! He only saw emergency admissions on his two official ward rounds, although there was one exception on one particular Saturday afternoon.

On that specific occasion, the Windsor Hospital chaplain, an erstwhile Geigy research chemist, had been admitted suffering from pneumonia complicated by agranulocytosis – the consequence of ten years of intermittent self-medication with Phenylbutazone (Butazolidin) for non-specific muscular aches and pains.

Dr Lister had come over essentially to ensure that the patient received the dignity and privacy afforded by a side room!

The outlook was deemed to be hopeless, but nonetheless I was instructed to contact Dr Lister immediately if there was any significant change in the patient's condition.

At some time between three and four o'clock on Sunday morning, the night sister contacted me to say that the chaplain had died, and would I come down to certify his death, so that the nurses could lay him out and have his body taken to the mortuary.

Having confirmed death, I found myself in a quandary.

Should I at this very point in time telephone Dr Lister and convey the grim news?

Maybe in the full light of day, and with my brain in gear, I would have waited, but instead I asked the switchboard to put me through to Dr Lister's home.

The phone rang for a while, and eventually the receiver was lifted.

A nondescript grunt came from the other end.

I unburdened myself as succinctly as possible.

There was a long audible silence, which was followed by a tirade of abuse, admonishing me for having unnecessarily disturbed his sleep.

51

Sometime later I wondered what his reaction might have been had I waited a few hours longer and missed him, because his frenetic daily work schedule made his whereabouts quite unpredictable.

At least, armed with the information he had so ungratefully accepted, he would have been able to contact the relatives personally and give the impression that he had actually been there when the poor chaplain had breathed his last.

Dr Lister went on to become the Linacre Fellow at the RCP!

In those days almost all the junior doctors at the hospital lived in, and paid a substantial sum from their meagre salaries for board and lodging. We were a motley bunch, congregating in the doctors' mess in between calls to attend the sick.

Continuity of care was self-evident and paramount.

We shared confidentialities and worked together for the benefit of our patients. In effect, this larger team ran the hospital without much need for the supercilious advice from the absentee Consultant staff.

For example, when we became thoroughly dissatisfied with the quality of the hospital food, our mess president informed the Hospital Secretary that in future we would be taking lunch between noon and 2.0 pm at the 'Feathers' – a hostelry about a mile up the road.

Within twenty four hours our demands were met, and our undivided service to patients returned to normal!

After four years in England I spent six years in Glasgow where the Consultant played a much more 'hands on' approach towards 'his' patients, but when it came to accepting responsibility for a patient who had died in unexplained circumstances, the Consultant was nowhere to be found!

This situation occurred one weekend when I was 'on call'.

The patient had come by ambulance to the Casualty Department. He was emaciated and covered in body lice. After gowning up I carefully examined the patient. The salient clinical finding was some crepitations (fine crackles) in his lungs. After taking some blood and entering these details in the patient's case notes, I asked the PRHO to arrange a chest x-ray, but the radiographer refused to allow her equipment to become contaminated before the patient had been deloused!

Because there was no such named facility in the hospital, the PRHO decided on his own bat to get an ambulance to take the patient to the infectious diseases unit at Robroyston Hospital, but on the way there the patient died.

The case was reported to the office of the Procurator Fiscal (PF), and several months later I was called as a witness. The PRHO, who should have been called, had in the meantime gone to find his fortune in the USA!

On the day of the inquest I had to wait for several hours in a dark foreboding corridor outside the chamber, whilst the PF interrogated the other witnesses.

When I found myself in the witness box, the PF seemed to me to be an unfriendly monster of a man sitting there in his official robes.

He asked me why I had not diagnosed pneumonia, when the Pathologist's report had identified that as the cause of death.

I offered my excuses. The PF nodded, and I was excused.

Outside the chamber I was taken to the cashier who paid me for the time I had spent in the building, and that was the end of it.

The Press had a field day with the PF's concluding remarks.

Professor Goldberg, who had been the Consultant 'on call' on the day in question, wasn't mentioned, nor Willy Walker, who had sent the patient to his death, but the details of how the patient had become a lodger in his own tenement and starved to death by his cohabiting son-in-law's family, became the real headlines.

At least the Scottish equivalent of the English Coroner's Court knew how to gather all the information and not make a pig's ear of it!

When I returned to England in a more senior capacity, it was the senior registrar who took on that 'hands on' role, with the Consultant still very much in the background.

This was the *modus operandi* which would persist for another couple of decades.

Another feature of hospital staffing in the 60s was the way in which PRHO and SHO posts were slotted into the system.

Almost all of these posts started on either 1st January or 1st July, and since their duration was six months for PRHOs and one year for SHOs, if sickness struck a junior member of staff, it was virtually impossible to find an appropriately qualified locum to hold the fort.

This situation played into my hands in 1962 while I was waiting to resit the O&G part of the Cambridge finals exam.

In 1962 the Cambridge final medical examination results were not due to be published until about ten days after 1st July. That meant that most Cambridge graduates applied for and were provisionally appointed for some of those forthcoming vacancies. Consequently for just over one week these 'medical students' would be working without the appropriate licence.

I fell into that category and started my first PRHO Surgery job on 1st July, only to find out after working for over a week in that post that I had passed Medicine and Surgery but failed O&G.

One might have thought that my current job, being in Surgery, would be OK, but one had to pass all three components in order to receive temporary registration from the GMC.

Thus, at the beginning of August I was out of work and would have to wait another five months before resitting the O&G part of the final MB examination.

However, as luck would have it, in September 1962 the O&G SHO at a neighbouring hospital had to undergo appendectomy for acute appendicitis, and was deemed unable to resume his job for four weeks.

The hospital managers searched high and low for a locum and finally, in desperation, asked me to fill that post!

Naturally I agreed, but the O&G Registrar was unhappy because he would be expected to cover my duties, thereby making his workload virtually continuous day and night for four weeks.

Management waived the usual precautions and just asked the Consultants to cover my activities when I was 'on call' (1:2), not that there was much chance that they would actually make the effort!

This was good experience for me and helped to fill the gaps in my O&G knowledge and prepare me for the retake of O&G in December, but maybe not so good for patient safety!

My first experience of using forceps came in the early hours of the morning. The mother had become exhausted and unable to make the final effort to deliver the baby's head, which was already presenting itself at the perineum. Under normal circumstance the doctor would apply forceps and help the baby out.

I hadn't the foggiest idea of which way round to attach the forceps and although the midwife would have been able to do the job perfectly competently herself, she was not 'allowed' to use forceps. Thus with the verbal encouragement of the midwife, I not only succeeded to apply the forceps correctly but also apply the necessary level of traction in the correct direction and achieve a very satisfactory result.

In a way that was child's play, but a week later there was a very different scenario.

A young woman, who was in the last trimester of her first pregnancy, had developed pre-eclampsia and was admitted for blood pressure control.

Soon after admission she started to have epileptic convulsions.

This was a serious emergency.

Because no Consultant was available, the O&G Registrar decided to perform an emergency Caesarean section.

An anaesthetist was called from the nearest hospital (King Edward VII Hospital in Windsor), and I was instructed to administer a rectal infusion of Avertin (Bromethol) to control the fits and hopefully reduce the blood pressure.

Shortly afterwards the patient was taken to the operating theatre.

The anaesthetist – the only Consultant in the operating theatre – was unhappy about the high blood pressure and gave the patient additional medication to control it.

Everything seemed to be going according to plan.

The 34 week old baby was delivered but, without adequate neonatal care on hand, died shortly afterwards.

As the incision in the abdominal wall was being sutured, the anaesthetist went very pale.

The patient's blood pressure had plummeted like a stone and had become barely recordable. He summoned Consultant backup from Windsor, and about half an hour later Dr Lister and his medical Registrar appeared on the scene.

By this stage the patient was moribund.

Dr Lister left his Registrar to call the shots, but she was an indecisive person with an apparent inferiority complex and, apart from ordering the administration of more Noradrenaline, when there were no accessible peripheral veins, her contribution was minimal.

The patient's heart 'stopped'.

There was no defibrillator!

The O&G Registrar drew the line at opening the chest and performing manual cardiac massage.

A half-hearted attempt was made at CPR (Cardio-Pulmonary-Resuscitation).

The patient was declared dead.

The husband, who had just arrived and was waiting in the corridor, was allowed into the theatre to find his dead wife and baby and a rather sheepish looking collection of doctors.

Today, that situation would have been managed very differently. In 1962 that was par for the course, when the cost of an appropriate level of risk management was left in the lap of the gods!

10

The Real Carers

It is easy to imagine that doctors run the show in hospitals, but without the nurses, our hospitals would fall apart.

Nurses provide the essential oil which lubricates the smooth running of the wheels of healthcare, and without them the system would grind to a standstill.

For as long as history has been recorded, it has been the womenfolk who have cared for the children and the members of the larger family, and when old age began to nibble away at the bodies of their elders, it was the woman's lot to add them to their burden of care.

It took the Crimean War, in 1854, to shake the British Establishment out of their complacent attitude towards the delivery of healthcare.

Florence Nightingale is remembered for her analysis of the filthy conditions in which the wounded were usually left to die, and her persistent petitioning of those in power to change the way in which hospitals were run, but it was the Jamaican, Mary Seacole, who inspired the nation by her feats of selfless ministrations to those wounded on the battlefield.

In 1860 the Nightingale Nurse Training School opened at St Thomas's Hospital in London.

In 1887 the British Nurses Association was created, and by then more hospitals had set up their own school of nursing and were applying Florence Nightingale's principles to train their own staff. In this environment, in exchange for lectures and clinical instruction, students provided the hospital with two or three years of skilled free nursing care.

In 1908 the first meeting of the National Council of Trained Nurses of Great Britain and Ireland was held in London.

During the First World War 10,500 nurses were enrolled.

In 1916 the Royal College of Nursing (RCN) was founded, and in 1919 the Nurses Act established the General Nursing Council and a register of all State Registered Nurses (SRN).

In 1940 the qualification of State Enrolled Nurse (SEN) was formally recognised after having completed two years of nurse training, but these nurses could not carry any of the responsibilities of their SRN counterparts.

In 1967 the Salmon Report proposed the development of nursing to include the management of hospitals

In 1972 the Briggs Committee suggested a move to degree preparation of nurses, and that nursing practice be based on research.

In 1983 the Griffiths Report established general management in the NHS, largely taking leadership away from nurses and doctors.

In the same year, the United Kingdom Central Council for Nursing, Midwifery and Health Visiting set up a new professional register with four branches (mental health, children, learning disability and adult) reflecting former types of training and qualifications: Registered General Nurse, Enrolled Nurse (General), Registered Mental Nurse, Enrolled Nurse (Mental), Registered Nurse for the Mentally Handicapped, Enrolled Nurse (Mental Handicap), Registered Sick Children's Nurse, Fever Nurse, Registered Midwife and Registered Health Visitor.

Right up until this time nurses in training were treated as apprentices. They paid nothing for their training, and received a small emolument to reflect their contribution to the care of patients in the hospital.

In 1986 the government launched Project 2000, which proposed to make nursing a university based diploma, and signal an end to hospital based schools of nursing.

Nurses would then have to pay fees to train as a nurse, although government sponsored grants would still be available.

2002   Nurses were enabled to prescribe medication
2004   RCN voted to make nursing a university degree.
2009   All nursing courses in UK become degree level.

The scope and status of nursing has changed since the days of Florence Nightingale and Mary Seacole.

The nurses who were recorded as part of the, 'Memories of Nursing' project, often practiced before the full professionalization of nursing had taken place. They trained in an apprenticeship model with little power or reward. However they often remembered the standards of care at that time with pride; the responsibility they were afforded with acceptance; and their rich, varied experiences with fondness.

As a medical student, in my first year of clinical experience at Barts, the ward wasn't just a place for corralling patients, but a micro-community with the ward sister as the queen bee at its head. She controlled everything starting with the care of the patients, to the wellbeing and education of her nurses, and the behaviour of the junior doctors and medical students, and last but not least she was the guiding light of the Consultant in charge.
For medical students, she could be your benevolent aunt or your nemesis!
In those days the medical students were the ward phlebotomists. Our task was to take blood from any patient identified by the PRHO, and start as soon as the nurses had finished their handover from the ward sister. This debriefing took place at the nursing station, which comprised a desk butted up against the central partition that divided the ward into two halves. The nurses were gathered around the ward sister whose back was towards the doors which separated the ward from the corridor, but leaving enough space for a trolley bearing a patient to pass without difficulty.
On my first day I arrived a little too early, entered the ward and then stood quietly while Sister Lawrence, a big woman, continued to engage with her flock.
One of the nurses caught my eye and I winked back, or did I gesture to her?
What I had not realised was that there was a mirror in front of Sister Lawrence – basically to act as the hidden eye in the back of her head. So when she had finished her task, she swivelled round in her chair and confronted me like a battleship with its 16 inch guns blazing.
It was a lesson which I never forget!

The transition, which has taken place in nursing since then, has not all been positive, but the need for caring, compassionate and competent nurses remains as important as ever.
In the hospital setting, the most important nurses were still the ward sisters, but advancement in nurses' careers was difficult without becoming a teacher, a manager, a specialist nurse practitioner or most recently, taking on the role of a Nurse Consultant. These jobs are in effect a way of staffing the NHS with lower paid appointees than would have been possible had they been doctors or career managers.

District Nurses were a bit different, because they remained as dedicated carers.

Once a nurse – always a nurse.
Once an academic – always an academic!

Two nurses from the old school stand out in my memory.

In recent times, the Deputy Director of Nursing at our DGH was a Welsh nurse with whom I crossed swords on a number of occasions. However, despite her exalted position in the hospital, she could often be seen in A&E with her sleeves rolled up and wearing a plastic pinny. The other nurses found this a bit intimidating despite the fact that she was working face to face with the patients, and not interfering with the roles of the senior A&E nurses. She went on to become the Director of Nursing at the General Hospital in Carmarthen.

In 1964, I was an SHO at the Wilson Hospital in Mitcham. The Matron could at times, when there was a shortage of nurses on the female medical ward, be seen doing menial tasks like handing out and collecting bedpans.

I asked her why she did not do the more responsible jobs on the ward instead, such as doing the drug round.

Her reply was simple.

She was not up to date with all the advances in medicine since she had been a ward sister, but she still knew how to care for patients!

Well, beat that!

Where in the caring professions do the doctors feature?

Psychiatrists – those who deal with the really mad and the mentally disturbed.
Surgeons – doctors with great manual dexterity and the ability to see human anatomy in three dimensions, giving them the ability to find and remove the foreign body, excise the uninvited guest and repair a faulty bit of the body's infrastructure.
Physicians – who play with random associations to make a diagnosis, but who still have to rely upon largely unscientific modes of treatment.
Pathologists – who attempt to apply today's science to solve yesterday's healthcare issues.

11

Playing God

The original Hippocratic Oath was a long convoluted list of rules which medical practitioners were obliged to follow, although I cannot actually remember ever having signed any document agreeing to abide by these rules.

However, the main tenet was, 'Do no harm'.

Therefore a doctor attempting to cut short the life of a patient would be viewed as breaching that oath, in addition to having in effect committed manslaughter or murder.

The doctor's power over the life or death of a patient is a multi-edged sword, and no matter how one might think up a legitimate excuse to 'commit murder' under the guise of relieving a patient of suffering, there remains a certain element of guilt attached to one's actions.

We may readily have a pet animal 'put down' under the guise of relieving the animal's suffering, but in reality it is our 'suffering', watching our pet endure a 'painful' illness, that we are actually relieving!

Applying the same action to a patient would be classed as euthanasia, but in the UK euthanasia is illegal, even when the patient provides a signed statement authorising the doctor to end their life.

The way round this impasse is either to withdraw life support or just wait for nature to 'take its course', despite the fact that we are in effect allowing the patient to be harmed.

Of course there are classical examples of doctors overstepping the mark and wilfully ending a patient's life for personal financial gain.

In 1957 Dr John Bodkin Adams was accused of murdering a patient who had made him a beneficiary in her will.

At that time I was a medical student, and there was great interest in the journalistic hyperbole attached to the case, but when he was acquitted one might have thought that nobody really cared.

When in 2000, Dr Harold Shipman became headline news for a similar type of malpractice, the newspapers had a field day, but he was successfully convicted of murder.

Between them they had probably prematurely ended the lives of several hundred patients using narcotics or barbiturates.

Dr Adams' trial failed on account of a lack of reliable witnesses.

Dr Shipman in that respect was less fortunate, because amongst other considerations, aggrieved relatives of his patients asserted that he had deprived them of their inheritances, and they were more than willing to come forward and testify.

He was found guilty, and sent to prison where he committed suicide still professing his innocence.

Dr Adams was subsequently convicted of prescribing irregularities and falsifying death and cremation certificates.

He was fined £2,400 plus costs of £457 (equivalent to about £70,000 in 2022) and was struck off the medical register, but was reinstated four years later and continued in private medical practice in Eastbourne for the next 22 years until he died at the age of 84.

In 1991 Dr Nigel Cox, a Consultant Rheumatologist, whose patient had begged him to end her life, was found guilty of murder, not because he had prescribed an excessive dose of narcotics for her intractable pain, but because he had, for no 'justifiable reason', intravenously administered a lethal dose of potassium chloride, when the other narcotic medication had failed to achieve its objective.

He had made no attempt to hide the fact or falsify the documentation, but a nurse decided to report the incident because, having apprised herself of the information, she could have been accused of having supported an offender.

Dr Cox was convicted of attempted murder and received a twelve month suspended sentence, but he was not struck off by the GMC. He was merely suspended from his hospital job for eighteen months, whilst being allowed to continue in Private Practice!

These were three cases of incontrovertible euthanasia, but with very different outcomes for the perpetrators.

In 1964 I was the medical SHO at the Wilson Hospital in Mitcham, Surrey. The junior medical staff comprised a medical SHO, a surgical SHO and a surgical Registrar. There was one medical Consultant and several surgical

Consultants who operated there, including an orthopaedic Consultant whose claim to fame was that he had been the first male medical student to study at the Royal Free Hospital in London.

My Consultant performed one ward round each week accompanied by a local GP, who would act as his locum during periods of leave, whilst I was in effect the most junior and also the most senior medical doctor on site.

It was quite a responsibility for someone with so little medical experience!

During the summer, a middle aged woman with a dense stroke was admitted. She was deeply unconscious with no discernible spontaneous or reflex muscular activity apart from the regular movement of her diaphragm and the rhythmic contraction of her heart.

The prognosis looked pretty bleak.

It was just a case of waiting for the inevitable, but that did not stop the nurses from giving her comprehensive nursing care, which they performed with great skill despite the patient's considerable bulk.

Medically speaking, she received no treatment. There was a vague hope that by not replacing body fluids, any associated cerebral oedema would be reduced and that in itself might help to raise her level of consciousness.

Forty eight hours later when my Consultant, Dr Friedlander, saw her, the outcome looked very gloomy indeed and, having up until then avoided speaking to the relatives, I found myself having to convey our pessimistic prognosis to her nearest and dearest.

Of her relatives, her daughter was the most upset. Her husband and son adopted a more pragmatic attitude, and after that first encounter did not come forward for subsequent updates.

Her daughter and one of her granddaughters were constant visitors and would sit at her bedside holding her hand with tears in their eyes. When visiting was over they would hang about waiting for me to give them moral support, but all I could do was to give them rather vague prognostications which only confirmed my ignorance.

After two weeks, some sort of active medical intervention was deemed necessary. Since she had no gag reflex, she needed intravenous fluids and that became my nightmare of finding suitable veins, in her well covered body, for the intravenous cannula. Once established, one hoped that further attempts to find a vein would be unnecessary, but the iv fluids were somewhat corrosive, and the dutiful turning of the patient by the nurses threatened to dislodge the cannula.

Sure enough, each drip site only lasted a few days before the cannula needed to be resited. The frequency with which the drip had to be resited was exacerbated after I had administered Parentrovite (one ampoule containing the B vitamins and the other vitamin C), which, even after dilution appeared to be highly corrosive.

Her emotional daughter and granddaughter continued to make my life a misery, for no matter how I tried to camouflage the inevitable outcome, they seemed to be praying for a miracle, whilst also appearing to wish that their traumatic experience could be brought to an end.

When the patient started to exhibit Cheyne Stokes respiration, I confidently predicted that the end was nigh.

Once again I was to be proved wrong.

Frequently her daughter asked if her mother was suffering, and whether there was anything I could do to alleviate her distress. She looked pleadingly into my eyes, but that was all.

The ward sister, who was a rather excitable Maltese woman, complained that the nurses' backs were taking a punishing from the two-hourly turning of the patient.

She was right, but what could I do?

It was as if the clockwork mechanism in the patient's brain stem had gone into autopilot, and nothing short of an act of God would put an end to the misery that her nearest and dearest appeared to be suffering.

Then rightly or wrongly I took the matter into my own hands.

If God would not do the right thing, then maybe I should step forward and resolve the issue for all concerned.

The plan was quite simple.

When the regular injection of Parentrovite was due, I planned to take a syringe loaded with potassium chloride.

The ampoules were there in the clinical room, along with the syringes and all the other iv paraphernalia.

There was no requirement to prescribe the potassium chloride, because it wasn't kept in the drugs cabinet.

Just behave in the usual way so as not to raise any suspicions.

I drew the curtains around the patient's bed, attached the syringe containing the lethal dose to the cannula, injected the potassium chloride and then slowly followed that with the diluted Parentrovite.

After a short while the patient stopped breathing.

I listened to her chest and could hear no heartbeat.

Her pupils started to dilate and then became fixed.

I collected the syringes together and left her bedside without pulling back the screens.

The syringes and needles were disposed of in the usual way, and I made an entry in the case notes to document the administration of Parentrovite.

I left the ward and went for lunch.

A short while later I received a call from the ward to tell me that the patient appeared to have 'passed away'.

I dutifully returned to the ward, and confirmed the death so that the nurses could start to lay the patient out.

However, there remained one possible snag which I had not taken into account.

There was a bizarre arrangement between the senior lab technician, the Coroner's Officer and the Pathologist at St Helier Hospital in Carshalton, whereby the lab technician usually reported all deaths at our hospital to the Coroner's Officer.

He was certainly overstepping the mark, but there was something in it for him, because that lab technician, with the compliance of the Pathologist, collected small samples of brain which he used to manufacture the reagent used to test for syphilis, and which he sold to other laboratories.

The Pathologist received the fee for performing the Coroner's post mortem.

The Coroner's Officer (a policeman) seemed to be no more than a patsy!

Fortunately for me, the senior lab technician was on holiday, and the other lab technician played no part in this charade.

So I was able to complete the death certificate, giving the cause of death as bronchopneumonia secondary to a cerebral thrombosis.

It had all been too easy!

At visiting time that afternoon I gave my condolences to the patient's daughter and granddaughter and handed them the death certificate.

The patient's daughter had already seen her mother's body in the hospital's chapel of rest. The body had no blemishes on it thanks to the assiduous nursing care, although both forearms were horribly scarred with bruising and thrombosed veins resulting from my frequent attempts to resite her iv drip.

Her daughter was composed, despite the ever present tears in her eyes. However these were not tears of anguish but tears of joy.

She looked steadfastly into my eyes and asked if her mother had suffered as her life ebbed away.

I reassured her that it had been a peaceful end.

She took my hand and squeezed it very tightly.

She really wanted to believe that on this occasion I had been telling the truth.

That was the end of this saga until a couple of years later when I was a Medical Registrar at Mile End Hospital in Stepney, where a middle aged West Indian lady had been admitted with a similarly dense stroke. The only difference was that she had not lost her gag reflex and therefore nutrition and fluids could be administered by a nasogastric tube.

The ward sister and her deputy were relatively young Irish girls – a devout catholic, and a lapsed catholic – but dedicated nurses nonetheless.

As the weeks passed there appeared to be little change in the patient's condition. I wondered how long it would be before I would be signing her death certificate.

Then, after about two months, the patient had what appeared to be an epileptic fit, and from then onwards she slowly recovered and eventually left hospital with very little disability!

Had I prematurely pulled the plug from that other patient in Mitcham?

Had I been less impatient, could she also have recovered?

Playing God isn't without having a future cross to bear!

12

Outlawing Criticism

In 1965, when I became a Medical Registrar at Mile End Hospital in Stepney, it took a while to understand the curious way in which patients were admitted.

From 9.00am to 5.00pm requests for admission were handled by the Hospital Secretary, and he admitted everything regardless, until all the beds were full. These requests came from GPs or the London Bed Bureau. For the next sixteen hours the resident Registrars took over that role.

One soon got to know which GPs would tell you a packet of lies in order to get a patient admitted, and how the Bed Bureau would try to persuade you to accept a patient who was not living in your local community. The main problem was that stroke patients in particular could occupy a bed for months, and if they lived outside one's locality they were very difficult to discharge. So with every request from the Bed Bureau we asked two questions before becoming involved – who was the patient's GP, and where did the patient live?

Within the hospital there were other problems and in particular the inability of those working at the coalface to influence performance and policies. Those at the top did not appear to have the humility to accept that they neither had any idea of what was happening at the workface, nor had the will to improve the system.

Long before professional managers took over the running of the NHS, inter-consultant rivalry and their inflated egos were not up for criticism by junior medical staff, even when mismanagement compromised the care of patients.

In 1966 I found myself with my head in the lion's mouth.

At that time there were three medical Consultants, but only two of them were part of emergency 'on call' rota. These two Consultants, Dr Sears and Dr Dolphin rarely spoke to each other, and viewed the other's activities with hostility.

I worked for Dr Dolphin, an Irishman with a wealth of experience which he readily passed on to his junior staff.

Dr Sears had the exalted title of Physician Superintendent, and held a key role on the hospital management committee. He gave the impression of a doctor who thought he ought to have been on the staff of a teaching hospital, but nonetheless enjoyed the privacy of his personal hospital accommodation to entertain any nurse who was up for it. He also had a penchant for female PRHOs whom he would appoint in preference to any male applicant.

The 1:2 duty rotas meant that the team on duty on Friday night would get the following weekend off duty until the following Monday morning. Conscientious junior doctors knew that Friday night's admissions usually required several hours to complete and make safe before the weekend team took them over, but that meant that their weekend leave often did not start until after midday.

Dr Sears' team usually left before these tasks had been completed and that made my weekend unnecessarily onerous, because Dr Dolphin forbade anyone other than his Registrar to see patients on Dr Sears' wards!

On the Saturday afternoon of this particular occasion I received a call from the sister of Dr Sears male ward, asking me to countersign a prescription for morphine which had been ordered over the phone by Dr Sears' PRHO during Friday night. The sister also added that the patient was looking a bit poorly.

When I arrived on the ward I found a grey looking patient fighting for breath and suffering from pulmonary oedema, but there were no notes made by Dr Sears' PRHO, and the report of the night staff in the ward nursing register recorded that the doctor 'on call' had not seen the patient, but had given a verbal instruction to the nurse in charge to administer 10mg of morphine.

After examining the patient, seeing to his medical needs and writing up his case notes, I rather foolishly wrote a scathing addendum in which I admonished the unprofessional actions of this PRHO and the apparent lack of appropriate supervision.

On the following Monday morning, whilst completing the ward round with my Consultant, I received a phone call telling me to report to the Physician Superintendent.

At that point I apprised my boss of that Saturday afternoon's debacle.

To my surprise, he was greatly amused.

Dr Dolphin seemed to greet this news as part of a point scoring competition.

72

In fact he commended me on my action.

Later that day I had an audience with Dr Sears.

He was livid and outraged with my having used the patient's case notes to air my disapproval.

In that he was justified, because clearly I should have written my complaint separately and sent the missive straight to Dr Sears, but since previous complaints had gone unanswered, I had felt justified in using this means.

I didn't mind being told off, but Dr Sears added a threat in which he clearly spelled out his intention to see that I did not get short-listed for another medical post in London.

During the last two months of that appointment I applied for a number of teaching Hospital Registrar posts in London, but was uniformly unsuccessful.

I contacted the Postgraduate Dean, but he gave me little reassurance.

In desperation I applied for a vacant Medical Registrar post at Glasgow's Western Infirmary (one of its two Teaching Hospitals), and was appointed!

Maybe I should thank Dr Sears for his efforts, because the next six years in Glasgow was the best period in my junior doctor experience!

As top down management became the norm, those at the bottom of the pile could quickly become the scapegoats when anything did not go according to plan.

These managerial bullies had no truck with whistle blowers.

If you rocked the boat, you could be fired and carry with you a stigma which would make you virtually unemployable in the NHS.

The NHS had become the domain for wielding the big stick, and no place for the carrot.

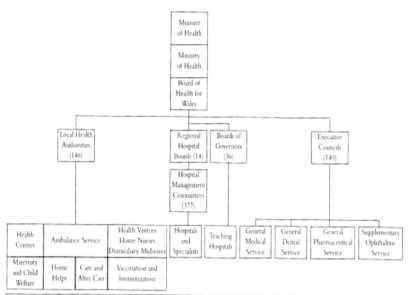

Source: C. Webster, The National Health Service: A Political History (Oxford, Oxford University Press, 1998), p21.

England & Wales Healthcare Scenario before 1974

PART IV

Evolution 1975-1995

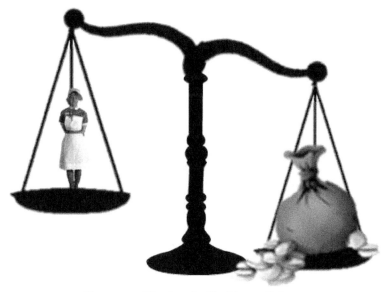

Commerce Tipping the Healthcare Balance

13

Taking Responsibility for the Service

The security of being appointed to a, 'job for life', is something that few employees can enjoy, but in the NHS, obtaining a GP or Hospital Consultant post usually meant just that – barring any serious misdemeanours.

In the summer of 1975, I attended for interview at the headquarters of the NE Thames Regional Health Authority in Eastbourne Terrace. I was one of three candidates for the vacant post of Consultant Physician at the St Helena Hospital Group in Colchester.

The appointment was 'Fulltime' but the successful candidate had the option of taking a 'Part Time' contract with a variable number of sessions to engage in Private Practice.

The specialty interest of the candidates was not of importance to the Regional Board, but had influenced the decision of the local representative on the interview committee, who made it clear who was their preferred candidate.

Maybe that had something to do with my appointment, but it was reassuring to know that the local community hospital still pulled the strings.

There was however a curious proviso in the terms of the contract. The Regional Board still had the authority to deploy the successful candidate to other parts of the NE Thames Region if the necessity were to arise.

I had about three months in which to work my notice as a Senior Registrar and also find accommodation for my family within ten miles of ECH.

My first impressions were like looking at the future through rose tinted spectacles. Colleagues were welcoming and supportive, although in one sense there was a feeling that one was having unpopular batons being passed down to the person who had just become the lowest common denominator, and the prime example was the almost immediate nomination as the next Secretary of the Medical Division – an onerous job with a smidgeon of kudos.

There was also an ambiance of generosity.
I discovered that new appointees had a once in a lifetime opportunity to be gifted a piece of equipment which could enhance the performance of their department and the experience of patients.
Aladdin's Cave was alluring, but there was a financial limit to any request.
After several weeks of cogitation, and an opportunity to discover the real handicaps of providing an Endocrinology Service in the sticks, I requested the purchase of an apparatus which could measure osmolality on samples of blood and urine.
At that time the chemical laboratory had to send such samples for the measurement of osmolality to a laboratory in Newmarket, and it took about a week to get a result.
This was totally unacceptable when it came to differentiating between the uncommon condition of diabetes insipidus, and the rather more common condition of psychogenic polydipsia. The defining test was the 'water deprivation test', which required close observation and frequent measurements of blood and urine osmolality, whilst the patient became increasingly dehydrated.
A patient with diabetes insipidus could become seriously unwell if the test was prolonged beyond the point when the diagnosis was apparent, and without a laboratory on site able to provide results within the hour, exposing patients with suspected diabetes insipidus to this diagnostic procedure was unethical.
The alternative was to refer such patients to the nearest Teaching Hospital, and in this case that was my *alma mater*, St

Bartholomew's Hospital in London – involving a whole day and a 130 mile round trip.

Our laboratory could not justify spending £1,000 of their capital budget on a piece of apparatus which would spend most of the year in a cupboard, but they were happy to carry out the tests if someone else bought the equipment.

In 1975 the paperwork entailed was minimal once our Medical Executive Committee had agreed to fund my introductory gift.

Twenty years later, similar requests for equipment or staff, had to fulfil the rigours of a 'Business Case', and would then spend months shuttling through a hierarchy of managers and committees before the order was actually placed and the money eventually released!

The success of a Business Case was driven predominantly by the aspiration of reducing future expenditure. The provision of a better service to patients played an almost insignificant part in this decision making process!

Audit

Apart from off the cuff improvements to the service, one could also use audit to highlight deficiencies, and recommend change.

In 1975, the birth of Area Health Authorities (AHAs) as an additional layer of management, ostensibly to improve efficiency and patient management, came with a subplot of using medical audit to justify changes in healthcare delivery.

In NE Essex our AHA included an energetic Medical Director, who had a bee in his bonnet about Diabetes Services. He had audited the hospital deaths attributable to diabetes mellitus and came to the conclusion that Colchester had a particularly bad record. I challenged his assertion and asked him to produce the evidence.

Over the next months he provided us with brief case summaries for each of the 43 patients he had identified.

In order to test his conclusions, I set up an evening meeting at our Postgraduate Medical Centre (PGMC) to which I had invited about a dozen doctors including medical registrars, GPs and Consultants. The task for each participant was to decide, from the thumbnail medical histories, how they would complete each death certificate.

The outcome of this audit was to accept diabetes as the main cause of death in each case, if there was agreement by ⅔ of the participants.

In only six cases did the participants agree that diabetes had been the main cause of death!

The Medical Director went away to lick his wounded pride, but diabetes came up again a few years later.

In the 1980's our Medical Division requested Management to appoint a Diabetes Nurse Specialist.

This request had been precipitated by the need to change all our insulin dependent patients to the new U100 insulins, instruct them in the use of the new plastic disposable insulin syringes, and the monitoring of blood glucose levels using testing strips! Achieving that educational enhancement for hundreds of patients, who were attending our hospital diabetes clinic, threatened to overwhelm the service.

However the critical issue, for the Director of Finance, was our assertion that this appointment would reduce hospital admissions. In his eyes that meant the number of staffed hospital beds could be reduced with an attendant reduction in expenditure!

When we audited the impact of the Diabetes Nurse Specialist on hospital admissions, we found that there had been no overall change!

A small reduction in adult admissions was countered by an increase in Paediatric and Geriatric admissions – predominantly because of serious hypoglycaemia, but management continued to believe that hospital services would in the long-term require fewer hospital beds, and reducing the number of hospital beds continued!

Interaction with Research & Ethics
This theme repeatedly came up for scrutiny during my professional life.

The audit of case notes was a pretty soft sort of self-appraisal except when it raised issues which needed a change of medical practice. Unfortunately problems tended to fester because doing things differently was complicated by the time available from colleagues who had commitments in Private Practice.

When the DoH mandated that every hospital trust should have a Research & Development (R&D) facility, our Medical Director asked me to be its chairman. This was accredited as an extra unpaid session, but if I so wished I could have dropped one of my clinical sessions.

I had no intention of doing that!

The Trust also had to employ a fulltime R&D scrutineer (a young lady with a science PhD) and give her secretarial support. More expense without any obvious benefit for patients!

I found myself looking at countless nursing related projects which were in effect audits addressing the issue, 'how are we doing?', rather than testing hypotheses. Buried amongst this confusion of paper were nagging issues around the ethical nature of these projects and therefore they also had to be submitted to the district ethics committee, on which I sat wearing my R&D hat, along with the hospital's representative appointed by our MAC.

She and I had a few laughs about their interpretation of the word, 'ethics'.

After I had retired, the local ethics committees from Colchester and Chelmsford were reconstituted in Witham (halfway between our two towns), but their committee was more concerned with risk assessment than ethics. I found myself having to renew the approval for my remaining research project, and then return to demonstrate that the volunteer could neither slide off the equipment nor be electrocuted! Quite simple!

Ethics has another face outside of medical practice.

In the 1980's a newly appointed colleague complained to me that our local AHEM had deliberately delayed the approval of a 'research' project which he had submitted, in order to get his own project to assume precedence, and therefore be able to take the soft money from the pharmaceutical company which was sponsoring this bit of post-marketing surveillance.

I unofficially looked through the exercise book in which our AHEM kept the record of submissions, and was horrified with the laxity with which he had performed his role.

I could not really duck the issue and raised it with our MAC chairman.

A few days later I found our Chief Operating Officer (CEO) waiting for me in my outpatient clinic. He persuaded me that he did not want this colleague to be seen to be punished for his misdemeanours, because that might attract unwanted outside attention, and he wanted to keep the matter out of the public eye. It was also clear that the original complainant had been leaned upon to withdraw his complaint. In return, our AHEM would step down.

I suppose this was the best possible result, but also underlined the way that the medical profession closed ranks when their honour was challenged.

However, this case involved another ethical issue.

Doctors are not supposed to accept 'hospitality' from drug companies, because this practice might induce us to prescribe that company's preparations, and even accept a financial inducement to do so. However, a way round these restrictions was to accept a fee, payable into the doctor's 'research fund' (thus avoiding it being taxed), in return for starting a patient on the drug company's drug. However, this 'research fund' might in effect be nothing other than a slush fund for departmental or personal 'entertainment'.

The immediate beneficiary was the patient, who did not have to pay for the first month or two of treatment.

The doctor benefitted by being paid when every anonymised surveillance form, which included such things as compliance and side effects, was returned.

The drug company benefitted, from this pump-priming procedure, especially when the medical condition being treated was likely to be a long-term affliction as in this case – 'essential hypertension'.

The principles of ethical behaviour did not benefit.

Some time after the dust had settled, a new a committee called 'The Three Wise Men' was set up, and to this committee any of our colleagues could lodge a medically related complaint.

The committee was composed of the Clinical Tutor, the MAC chairman and the Ethics representative – later that became me.

This committee could have prevented the subsequent cancer waiting time scandal, but being separate from Management, it had no teeth!

Back in the real world, daily life was still about getting one's head down and getting on with the day job.

Many of us continued to be buoyed up by the prospect of an all singing and dancing new hospital being built, although I had no idea just how long and how fraught that process had already become!

If I and my colleagues had had the advantage of seeing what was likely to happen over the next twenty years, we might have been less ready to accept what was being handed down by the politicians.

In that respect, I had failed.

Like most of my colleagues, I was too naïve to realise that the path which the NHS was following was being repeatedly diverted away from the real healthcare issues of service development and sustainability.

Bean counting had by then become the top priority.

14

Enhancing Hospital Infrastructure

Anyone who has had any experience in industry would tell you that in order to remain competitive it is necessary to invest some of ones' profits in the modernisation of the business. For the NHS that meant replacing obsolete hospital infrastructure with new or refurbished buildings. However, this was usually well beyond the amount of money given to each individual hospital for capital projects. Furthermore, the NHS was not a competitor, but a provider of an essential service.

Investment wasn't needed to make the NHS more competitive, but to make it more effective at delivering its services.

Then there was the construction industry to contend with.

When it came to hospital building contracts, big business soon realized that they had the NHS over a barrel. It was generally the case that any hospital construction would be charged at least double the rate per square metre than would apply to other types of public building contracts.

The building fraternity wouldn't have dared to have exploited the voluntary/charity hospitals in this way before 1948!

Healthcare isn't something which can be neatly packaged as a single entity. It covers a wide spectrum of different activities from the acuteness of sudden trauma or disease, to the care of the impoverished elderly and the dying.

It would have been very convenient if the NHS could have taken over the ownership and management of the whole of this mishmash, but charity and commerce tugged in opposite directions at the heartstrings of the community.

Why should people who could afford to look after their relatives, expect the exchequer to take on this responsibility? After all was said and done, long ago it would have been the family who looked after their relatives in their final years.

The idea that the NHS would look after you from cradle to grave was nothing more than a socialist slogan.

This was true in communist states, even though the level of care varied according to status.

The hard bit for the NHS was drawing the lines of demarcation between saving the lives of otherwise healthy people, and the endless prolongation of life.

Prior to 1948 there had been no significant operational or financial linkage between the various hospital healthcare facilities in NE Essex, but thereafter these facilities could be viewed as an operational whole and amenable to functional rationalisation, because the overarching landlord was the NHS. With over 14 different outlets in NE Essex performing a variety of functions spread over an area from Braintree in the west, to Clacton on the east coast, each facility was still being managed separately.

In regard to Colchester itself, a new management structure was implemented by the Regional Board.

The new committee was called the 'Colchester Group Hospital Management Committee'. It's Chairman and members were not elected by the local community, but selected and appointed by the Regional Board, which charged them with the responsibility of making best use of the local hospital infrastructure, which included:

> ECH built in 1820
> St Mary's Hospital (the local workhouse)
> The Isolation (Fever) Hospital at Mile End
> Colchester Maternity Home

Psychiatric services were at:

> Severalls Hospital
> Turner Village Hospital
> Essex Hall

There were some locally managed cottage hospitals at:

Clacton
Halstead
Harwich

Plus a tuberculosis sanatorium at:
Black Notley.

A London County Council rehabilitation centre in Clacton;
Passmore Edwards Home

A MOD facility:
The Military Hospital

Add to this a large number of care homes for the elderly and chronic sick, such as the 100 bedded Heath Hospital in Tendring, which were operated by the local authorities concerned, and funded out of local taxation, supplemented by the Department of Health's Community's budget.

With each facility having its own budget and management structure, this was not conducive of cooperation or amalgamation. Thus, although there was a rationale for centralization, there were many hurdles placed in the way of achieving that goal.

The central hospital in NE Essex was ECH, and their management was quite happy to use space in other parts of the patch to reduce the pressure on the limited number of beds at the centre of Colchester.

With the NHS footing the bill for this cross-over activity, nobody gave the matter further thought, despite the inefficiencies which accompanied the practice.

Within six months of the inception of the NHS, the Chairman of the Colchester Group Hospital Management Committee made a proposal, at the Regional Board's regular meeting with district Chairmen, to build a new hospital on a massive 42 acre green-field site behind the Colchester Maternity Home.

At that time this land was owned by Essex County Council.

The scheme would have entailed the establishment of a 900 bed hospital and become a modern centre of excellence outside

London (something which appealed to the Labour government's plan to reduce centralization within the capital).

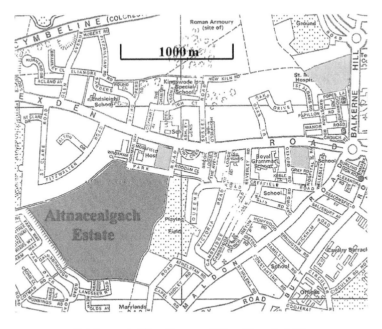

Colchester's First Proposed New Hospital Site

The Regional Board made a verbal agreement with Essex County Council, to earmark this site for the development of an NHS facility.

The Gynaecologists, who were being offered alternative accommodation for their gynaecology patients at St Mary's Hospital, saw this as a much better solution to the shortage of beds at ECH. It made sense to have all their staff concentrated in the same area, particularly when obstetric emergencies arose. Furthermore their private obstetric patients were also delivered at the Maternity Home. If the other specialties could be persuaded to join them in this venture, there would also be the possibility of closing some of the other hospital sites.

The optimism of Colchester's MAC, believing that they had favoured status at the Regional Board, was founded upon the ease with which they had already acquired a Radiotherapy

Department – something that in the pre-NHS era would have been impossible to finance from charitable donations.

However, they had overlooked the fact that the driving force behind that denouement had been the Director of the Radiotherapy Department at the London Hospital!

As it turned out, repeated vacillation by the County Council and indecision by the NETMRB left the building of the new hospital in limbo, and without the land actually being acquired by the NHS the prospect looked gloomy.

In 1951, the anti-socialist rhetoric used by the Tory Party, and the uncharacteristic agreement of Clement Atlee to get involved in the struggle between the Prime Minister of Persia and British Petroleum over the Persian government's nationalisation of their oil industry, persuaded the electorate that keeping a Labour administration in power would be a national disaster. The USA had already become obsessed with the idea that communism, or any form of socialism, would destroy the free-loading nature of capitalism.

Despite the Labour Party having successfully launched the 1951 Festival of Britain, Tory propaganda succeeded in downplaying everything that had been achieved by their opponents.

The gullible electorate swallowed the Tory misinformation, and voted in a Conservative Government.

Now the socialist revolution was well and truly over before it had had the time to hone its vision of healthcare into something that would be financially sustainable and uniformly acceptable to all parts of our diverse community.

However, the unfettered optimism of the Colchester Consultant body kept their dreams of a new hospital alive until 1954, when the County Council decided (without due consultation with the other parties) that the 42 acre Altnacealgach Estate behind the Maternity Home would be used for educational purposes.

As a result, between 1957 and 1965, three schools, the County High School for Girls, St Benedict's Roman Catholic School and the Philip Morant (comprehensive) School were built on that site.

Reading between the lines, the Department of Health was not in the business of purchasing more land, particularly when it had potential sites on their massive psychiatric land portfolio, so unless the local authority or the County Council were willing to barter this green field site for a similarly sized piece of NHS real-estate, the venture was dead in the water.

In 1948 land, which had been deemed surplus to immediate NHS requirements, was used for affordable social housing projects with the encouragement of the Minister of Housing, who coincidentally was also the Minister of Health – Nye Bevan.
After 1951, with the Conservatives firmly back in the saddle, any 'surplus' real-estate would be sold to the commercial sector for private housing schemes. Therefore unless the Tory Party could be persuaded to change their minds on social healthcare, we would have to wait in Colchester for the next Labour government, before our centralization programme could get off the starting blocks again.
The memory of being short-changed for political reasons lived on, but the delivery of healthcare in NE Essex could not wait.

Waiting lists for hospital outpatient appointments and non-acute surgical operations were becoming an embarrassment. These were addressed by capital investment on the various hospital sites and the recruitment of new staff. This gave the impression that we were coping with adversity (as we always had done), but this did not lessen the need for a new modern hospital and the potentially more efficient delivery of healthcare.
At this time ECH had 269 beds, but in spite of its ancient and in places dilapidated state, it offered the following services:

a.   General Medicine and Surgery
b.   Paediatrics

c.   Cancer & Radiotherapy
d.   ENT
e.   Dermatology
f.   Ophthalmology
g.   Gynaecology
h.   Pharmacy
i.   Radiology
j.   Haematology & Biochemistry Laboratories
k.   Private Patients

By March 1949, the waiting list for inpatient treatment at ECH had risen to 2,150. This demand seemed to have been in part due to patients who might otherwise have soldiered on without treatment, and in part due to GPs making hospital referrals for patients which they previously would have managed themselves.

The shortage of available beds at ECH was also compounded by the presence of a significant number of 'chronic sick' patients who had been deemed unable to be discharged home.

Sounds familiar!

There was a major outcry when an acutely ill patient, who had been taken to the Casualty Department at ECH, was in the process of being transferred to Clacton Hospital, and then died in the ambulance!

Red faces and the shuffling of items on committee papers provoked a kneejerk reaction.

It was claimed that the Isolation Hospital could provide up to 100 beds, but when push came to shove only 24 could actually be made available. However, before that could take place, the stigma attached to being a non-infectious patient in the 'Isolation Hospital' had to be addressed by changing the name of the hospital to 'Myland Hospital'!

With a little more thought, an additional 30 beds were added making a total of 54.

With the support of the local council, some chronic sick patients from ECH were transferred to Heath Hospital – the care home in Tendring.

The other change of usage was to open 16 surgical beds and a new operating theatre at St Mary's Hospital.

Additionally a generous offer was made by the Military Hospital to operate on male patients from the ECH surgical waiting list.

Further help was at hand with Black Notley Hospital getting the green light to provide extra accommodation for nurses on their site, so that some of their empty beds could be made available for patients from Colchester.

One might have argued that this was like sending good money after bad, when the long-term solution would have been to build the new hospital, but it was hoped that all this would contribute weight to our arguments rather than it becoming a millstone around our necks.

Just to add insult to injury, the NETMRB announced that our expenditure (the cost of delivering the service) during that financial year would be reduced by £60,000!

We argued that making savings on our budgeted costs of that magnitude would likely lead to staff redundancies and the closure of beds. Our protests fell on deaf ears, until Nye Bevan himself visited our area and countermanded that dictat!

Over the next twelve years similar adjustments and enhancements were made to accommodate more patients and recruit more medical and nursing staff, but increasing demands from the public and the development of new technologies meant that the chronic bed shortage never kept pace with demand, and unwieldy waiting lists became a source of disgruntlement, particularly if you had been on the waiting list for more than one year, and could not afford to 'go private'.

One might have expected with East Anglia, being a stronghold of the Tory Party, that successive Ministers of Health would have looked favourably on the needs of Colchester.

On a number of occasions it was reported that negotiations on building a new hospital had restarted, only to be told that these had come to nothing.

The distraction of the Suez Crisis, with the USA blackmailing Britain into a monetary black hole, meant that NHS capital developments stopped.

Making Enoch Powell, a man with no social conscience, Minister of Health, was another Tory cockup. He 'welcomed' foreigners to come and train as doctors and nurses, but expected them to return home to their native countries after qualifying. He had little idea of the need to retain such valuable resources!

In January 1962, the Government published a White Paper on the future NHS capital spending programme. In this ten year plan they identified £500 million to be spent on hospital infrastructure.

There were no details about how this money would be divided amongst the fourteen regions, but enthusiastic, probably overenthusiastic, reports were bandied about.

These included £5 million for an 800 bed new hospital in Colchester, and built at one of three proposed locations:

1. The MOD's Monkwick Artillery Ranges
2. The Severalls Hospital Site
3. The Turner Village Hospital Site

Thus we would be able to close ECH, St Mary's, Colchester Maternity, Black Notley, Halstead and Heath Hospitals – with enormous efficiency savings!

For those of us who had seen through previous government grand gestures, this was just a bit of political manoeuvring ahead of the next General Election.

Upbeat gestures like this were repeatedly verbalised over the next twelve months as Macmillan and his cronies tried to bury the Vassall and Profumo affairs, but these embarrassments still kept rocking the Tory boatload of Old Etonians, who were not renowned for their truthfulness let alone their social consciences.

In Colchester we already had approval from the NETMRB to spend almost £250,000 on specific projects, which included £150,000 to build a state of the art Radiotherapy Centre on the ECH site.

The London and Barts Hospitals had championed this development because their own departments had difficulty coping with the increasing use of deep radiotherapy treatment for cancer, and in this scenario long waits spelled reduced survival. That was in addition to the long journeys that sick patients had to travel in order to avail themselves of treatment. They were not concerned about the false logic of building this new service on a site earmarked for closure within ten years!

However, pipe dreams are only pipe dreams, and pragmatism was the name of the game.

Nonetheless, the future prospect of building a substantial hospital elsewhere in Colchester in order to centralise services remained on the back burner, although the prospect of using the MOD Monkwick Ranges had by then been dropped.

In 1964 the new Radiotherapy Centre was opened.

It had not been short changed.

Ground floor layout includes consulting rooms, examination rooms, offices and treatment rooms, the latter surrounded by barium blocks or dense concrete. Outpatients and inpatients are treated; a bedlift connects to the ward above

23-bed nursing unit on the first floor. Since some patients may be given fairly high radioactive dosages, all ward compartments are protected by 4 ft. high by 9 in. thick walls of dense concrete, with glazing above for easier supervision

Colchester's Radiotherapy Department in 1960

At about this time the Colchester Group Hospitals Management Committee, and the committee which had been overseeing the running of psychiatric services at Severalls Hospital, combined their efforts and planning activities to form the St Helena Group Hospital Management Committee.

The psychiatric component of this group added the following services to the melee:

a.   General Psychiatry at Severalls Hospital
b.   Electroencephalography/Physiology Service
c.   A Medical Psychiatric Ward
d.   Radiology

Additionally there were the Eastern Counties' *Institution for juvenile mental subnormality* at Turner Village Hospital, and the Eastern Counties' *Asylum for Idiots* at Essex Hall.

The inclusion of Severalls Hospital offered potential accommodation for some extra general medical and surgical activity, as well as being a possible site for the new hospital, with over 120 acres to choose from, and it was close to the A134 (Mile End Road) at its western boundary.

Just like the two other possible sites on the north side of the town, it already had all the essential services, including an on-site laundry.

Myland Hospital offered the next most promising site for future development, being surrounded by a considerable acreage of fields on which a new hospital could be built, before the need to find alternative accommodation for the NHS services already on that site. Furthermore the land bordering Mill Road was relatively flat.

Turner Village Hospital was the least suitable location, despite it being surrounded by farmland used by the inmates for occupational and recreational purposes. Additionally, the site was partially waterlogged, poorly drained, sloped steeply downwards towards the town, had a public footpath running through it, and was served by Turner Road, which was little more than a narrow tortuous lane, and the Borough Council had no intention of either closing or rerouting that public footpath!

However, for reasons which were hard to understand, the Turner Village site was temporarily preferred for any new general hospital development!

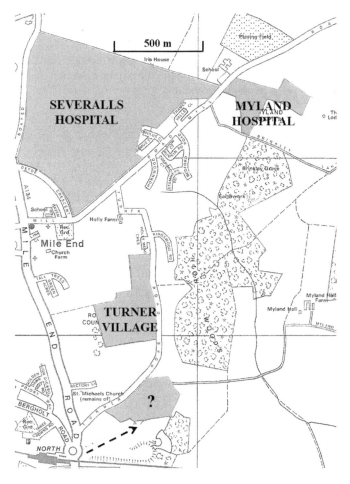

Hospital Sites North of the Railway in 1948

Any Health Minister concentrating on what would be best for the long-term delivery of healthcare in NE Essex, would not have chosen the Turner Road site, but the Ministry appeared to be more concerned with bean counting and lining the pockets of their capitalist colleagues, than the delivery of a sustainable healthcare service in Colchester!

The 1964 General Election spelled the death knell of the Tory's thirteen year rule. Their pre-election 10 year £500 million promise of capital investment in the NHS didn't convince the electorate, nor was the reminder, 'we never had it so good' in the 1950s, a promise that more of the same would revive the flagging economy.

Harold Wilson's Labour Party majority of only 4 seats in Parliament did not give him much room for lavish NHS spending.

Repeated submissions to Kenneth Robinson, the Minister of Health, by Colchester's Tory MP, Tony Buck, demanding that our new hospital project should be given priority, were met with evasive answers.

Then an 8,000 signature petition to prioritise the project was delivered to Kenneth Robinson, but with such a small proportion of the local population signing, this was unlikely to cut much ice.

In 1966 some confusion was added to the fray by the inclusion of another potential site for the new hospital. It involved land which was part of the Highwoods Country Park running parallel to the railway. This site would require a new access road from the railway station roundabout, but without further extension of this road, it would cut off access to Myland Hall and its farm.

It was also revealed that the NHS only owned the 17½ acres on which the Turner Village Hospital had been built, and that building on that site would require the purchase of an additional 19½ acres of farmland.

A public consultation was held and many objections were raised to both Turner Road sites.

Then the County and Borough Councils entered the ring, declaring that until decisions had been made about the future town plan and a new road network, further discussions were pointless.

In January 1968 a visit by Kenneth Robinson was scheduled in the hope that he could be forced into a corner, but at the last minute the Minister cancelled the visit.

97

About nine months later he did make the effort, but refused to take any questions!

However, it is worth remembering that at that time the annual budget for the whole of the NETMRB was £51 million, of which £6½ million was for capital projects. The estimated cost of building the new hospital in Colchester was about £7 million. Furthermore the £500 million capital funding promised by the Tory Party only amounted to £50 million per annum shared by 14 Regional Health Authorities. So £6½ million was quite generous, but totally inadequate for any major construction project, let alone keeping the existing infrastructure fit for purpose, and Colchester had already benefitted from major enhancements!

Additionally, the NHS policy of creating Regional Specialty Centres on existing hospital sites top-sliced the capital budget.

We had benefitted at ECH by getting a Radiotherapy Centre, Black Notley Hospital had become a Regional Orthopaedic Centre and Billericay Hospital a Regional Burns and Plastic Surgery Centre, although these were not the only Specialty Centres draining our region's capital building budget!

The building of new hospitals had barely been part of the previous Tory Party's thirteen years in office.

Just two were completed!

Since no privileged status for Colchester on the capital investment ladder was ever likely to make this Tory heartland return a Labour MP to Parliament, Harold Wilson needed to concentrate on winning back the Labour seats that had been lost in the 1951 General Election.

In Colchester the St Helena Group Hospital Management Committee continued to cherish the idea of building their new hospital, even if it meant waiting a bit longer and throwing more good money after bad as they tried to enhance local services and carry out backlog maintenance.

In 1966, when the Labour Party called a General Election and secured a massive 98 seat majority in Parliament, we became buoyed up once again.

The Turner Village Hospital site was finally chosen over all the other contenders, not because it was the best site for a new hospital, but because the site was the least attractive for future commercial development!

All sorts of suggestions, on how to combine our current services on the Turner Road site, were fantasized about, but nobody seemed to have remembered that the Severalls Hospital site would have been the most advantageous in the long run and, apart from the diminishing psychiatric workload, it had the Nurse Training facilities there.

Still there was no official statement about when the ball might start rolling again, nor in the interim did the NETMRB offer to pay for the necessary survey and architect's fees, or the cost of getting planning permission.

Whilst the Consultants supported the plans, they did not in fact move heaven and earth to lobby Parliament or their own professional bodies to do something about the impasse. Individual specialties made the case for their own slice of any future cake, and this often became a talking point at the Hospital Arms, the watering hole opposite ECH, but it was only talk and pipe dreams, and without some political clout that was likely to be as far as it would go.

In the 1970 General Election, the Tories were returned to power, but the Prime Minister, Edward Heath, had more on his plate than the needs of healthcare in Colchester.

Hope was revived in 1974 when the Conservative Party called a snap election, hoping to increase their majority in Parliament, but they lost the election, and it took Harold Wilson's Labour administration until 1978 to get our show back on the road.

Things really began to move again, and after the necessary land purchases had been made, and the Borough Council had given it the green light, no doubt the Labour Party thought they might have made sufficient impression upon the local population to return a Labour MP in the 1979 General Election.

This was a well tried Ministerial gambit, but it had been unsuccessfully tried by the Tories in the 1964 General Election, with their overblown promise of massive capital investment in the NHS.

Now the Labour Party wooed Colchester with a commitment to build their new hospital, but that horribly backfired, because the Tories, headed by Margaret Thatcher, were returned to power before any detailed plans had been drawn up.

15

Colchester's New Hospital

The journey of Colchester's redevelopment plan finally started during the death throes of Harold Wilson's Labour administration, but Mrs Thatcher's future union bashing, privatisation agenda was not going to be side-tracked by our plight, although perhaps she felt a sense of gratitude that Colchester had supported the Tory cause in spite of the Labour Party's promises. So the project went ahead, but with uncompromising Tory limitations.

There was never any consideration of what would be best for the local community, who after all would be the beneficiaries of the scheme.

In 1979, the Regional Board invited a medical representative from Colchester to attend a committee in London where all the decisions would be made, and accordingly, at a meeting of our MAC, the name of one of our anaesthetists was proposed for this task.

With nobody else prepared to devote any time to this important task, RGFG was elected *nem. con*!

At first sight this formality looked like a meaningful attempt at engagement with the needs of the local community, but it soon became clear that RGFG would be nothing more than a whipping boy.

There were weekly meetings over several months at the Regional Board's headquarters at Eastbourne Terrace in London, with the medical input to these meetings being orchestrated by two healthcare professionals, Dr Trevor Sussman, a surgeon who had given up surgical practice in 1970 in order to follow a career in Public Health, and Nurse Wooley, who had not witnessed life at the sharp end for a very long time. This pair was like caricatures of Jack Sprat and his wife, but the dominant partner was the larger than life Nurse Wooley, who had exchanged the life of a nurse for the theatrical forum of bossing people about.

Two young seemingly inexperienced architects, who had had little previous exposure to hospital construction, were given the task of cobbling together a workable plan.

When the MAC in Colchester were apprised of the fact that the budget for this project could not exceed £10 million, the reality of the situation became clear. This sum would never be enough to build a modern hospital capable of delivering a comprehensive medical service to the local community, let alone future proof it against any changing tide of medical practice.

The new hospital would be called a 'Nucleus' District General Hospital (DGH) to which the missing pods could be bolted on over the next decade.

By 1979 when the final plans were revealed, we found we had been saddled with a mirage, because no allowance had been made for the fact that with this DGH being built on the only relatively level part of the Turner Road site, these pods could not be simply 'bolted on'.

Perhaps, even at this late stage, we should have insisted on seeing what the hospital would have looked like when these missing bits had been added, but such detailed plans would have added more expense to the £10m which had already been accounted for!

We just had to accept the honesty and assurances of the Government's agents, when any fool knew that politicians were at best little more than twofaced dissimulators! Furthermore, and unbeknown to us at the time, this DGH module had already been deemed obsolete even before the diggers had moved in!

Had we been better informed, sufficiently outraged and properly motivated to challenge this political sledge hammer, we might have halted the process in its tracks and demanded that any new hospital development should be sited on the Severalls Hospital campus, which was already being depopulated in accordance with the other national master plan – to repatriate all but the most severely deranged psychiatric patients back into the community. Additionally the 120 acre Severalls Hospital site was level, unhampered by housing developments, which were beginning to smother the Turner Road area, and was already beautifully landscaped. In this way there would be no need to develop the site in a series of unsettling building projects.

It could have been all over and done with in one fell swoop, but that would just be a restatement of our previous aspirations!

Nonetheless, this was still the most logical way in which to develop healthcare in NE Essex!

Unfortunately, when it comes to providing the population with socially engineered healthcare, politicians suffer from short-sighted tunnel vision!

Thus we were lumbered, and without some genius finding a way to reconfigure the Turner Road site, future developments would more likely than not evolve into a mixture of randomly placed bits of Lego!

Long-term planning had never been part of any political party's strategy, because they knew only too well that with elections every five years, nothing was guaranteed.

The original 1945 long-term NHS vision of the Labour Party came to nought after only six years in office, and they had only three years to mould the NHS into shape, because they were ousted in the 1951 General Election, and remained in the doldrums for the next thirteen years – enough time for the Tory capitalists to wreak havoc with socialism.

How did the electorate judge the five years of Labour Administration from 1945-1951?

Were they swayed by a concerted Tory propaganda campaign which portrayed socialism as the next inevitable step to communism?

The USA was busy massaging the communist threat to the capitalist dreams of the average American citizen.

Was the Labour Party, which had disposed of the British Empire's greatest asset, India, to be trusted?

Pre-election rhetoric rarely gives a true assessment of what has been achieved, and in 1950 the NHS had only been in place for about 18 months.

For the Labour Party's parliamentary majority to have fallen from 146 to just 5 seats, tells one something about the vulnerability of our democratic electoral system.

The Tory hierarchy had been wounded but not disabled.

Britain had flirted with social democracy, but wasn't ready to marry into it.

Atlee called a snap election in 1951, hoping to regain that loss of trust, only for the Tories to win an overall majority of 17 seats despite polling fewer of the popular votes.

The fickle electorate had been bought by Tory propaganda.

1979 heralded the next eighteen years of Margaret Thatcher's Tory capitalist political agenda.

Investment in the health of the nation was never going to be part of Margaret Thatcher's game plan, but the thought of investing a small amount of capital for the purposes of local hospital centralization was tempting, if this lead to a reduction in running costs, and at the same time released NHS real estate to sell off to the Private Sector, along with selling off all the other nationalized industries that she could lay her hands on, and giving council tenants the right to purchase swathes of social housing.

What with annual North Sea oil revenues adding about £8 billion to the Treasury, one might have thought that Mrs Thatcher would lavish some of these riches on the NHS instead of reducing personal taxation.

You must be joking!

Back in Colchester, the doctors competed with each other to gain the best deal for their individual specialties.

Clearly there would be winners and losers and no guarantee that today's losers would become tomorrow's winners when the next phase of this development was initiated.

Colchester's DGH was opened by the Queen in 1985, but did she really realise that such royal occasions do not add any credibility to the process?

The accommodation for junior doctors had been poorly designed and had not been completed. It consisted of a collection of two storey bare unrendered breeze block buildings scattered around the north-west part of the site. They were damp, their roofs leaked, and in the winter the windows streamed with condensation.

Accommodation in the Siberian gulags was better than this!

These buildings should have been condemned, but it wasn't until Mike Pollard, the newly appointed CEO in 1995, who spent a few days living there himself, that they were bulldozed and proper accommodation was provided!

At about the same time the Borough and County Councils wanted to build a new northern approach road which would eventually link up with the A12 Colchester bypass, and to do that they would need the land on which these shacks had been built. It would also give the Council the opportunity to sell the land between this new road and Mile End Road for another housing development.

Capitalism, as ever, was always going to be the driving force in this agenda!

It would take another fifteen years after the DGH had been opened for most but not all of the major medical services that were missing to be added, and that was followed by the erection of various buildings, mostly prefabs, stuck on like pieces of Lego.

Long-term planning in the NHS had become a joke!

Parts of the Turner Road site, having been acquired by NHS Estates to build an inadequate new hospital, were sold off.

The 11.8 hectares (29.1 acres) of farmland to the south of Turner Village Hospital was sold in 2002 to the North East Essex Primary Care Trust (PCT) for the construction of a Healthcentre and new PCT headquarters. The remainder was sold to a property consortium to build a school and several hundred houses, which just added to the misery of the congestion in the poorly appointed road serving the hospital!

In due course the Essex Hall, Severalls and Myland Hospital sites were sold for housing, and the controversial site near the railway station was developed into a large retail park. St Mary's and Black Notley Hospitals were also sold for housing projects, and the Maternity Home became a Care Home.

The sale of NHS land continued unabating over the next five decades instead of using it for NHS purposes.

Between 2015 and 2018 a total of 3,627.1 hectares, i.e. 8,959 acres were disposed of in this way!

NHS Estates have other affairs which they might not be too proud of.

Starting in the 1962s, they 'oversaw' the building a number of new hospitals using building materials which have subsequently proved to have been of unproven suitability, and four of these hospitals were in East Anglia – the Queen Elizabeth Hospital, James Paget Hospital, the West Suffolk Hospital, and Hinchingbrooke Hospital. In each case cheap low density aerated concrete was used to form the ceiling/floor which separated the ground floor from the floor above.

Today that concrete is crumbling and posing a critical hazard that has required the insertion of a large number of steel supports, at great cost, in order to prevent the upper floor from collapsing onto the areas below.

However the worst part of this catastrophe is that NHS Estates and the DoH have not made any meaningful plans to provide alternative accommodation for patients in these districts, nor planned new properly constructed hospitals to replace these abominations.

The other revelation that came out of this saga was the attempt to sell off Hinchingbrooke Hospital to the Private Sector before its structural problem became critical.

Maybe that had been the hidden agenda for the other poorly built hospitals!

I suppose we in Colchester should be glad that we did not get one of those building experiments wished upon us.

Our fate was different, but equally unsatisfactory.

The disappointment of having Colchester's hospital development master plan cast aside once again by the Regional Board in the early 1970s had been a body blow but, rather than taking the bit between our teeth and working hard on a new plan, the Consultants withdrew into their world of private medicine, gaining solace from the homely way in which Private Practice was run and appreciated by all those patients who chose not to be part of any delusional NHS dream.

Thus the politicians, instead of seeing the NHS nurtured and enhanced to meet the growing population and the impact of new technology, just continued to fritter away the resources as the body of the beast was slowly being whittled down to the bone. The dismantling of healthcare seemed to have become the political priority, whilst the medical profession seemed to look the other way and lose the last vestige of credibility.

There were countless examples up and down the country of the cavalier way in which the politicians emasculated the health service, and the fate of Colchester typifies this *modus operandi*.

However, for the naysayers to declare the Colchester DGH as a fiasco would be to overlook its good points.

The hospital was like the Curate's Egg – 'very good in parts'.

Previously the Casualty Department at ECH, despite many upgrades, had been little more than a large cupboard with a few curtains separating the trolleys. The DGH offered a large dedicated Accident & Emergency (A&E) Department (the new brand name for the old Casualty Department), which was subdivided to deal with 'Resuscitation', 'Major' and 'Minor' emergency patients, and with its own dedicated x-ray facility for patients with fractures.

The old hospital's excuse for an Intensive Treatment Unit (ITU) had been a small area with a few trolleys situated by the entrance to the operating theatres. It was close to where the anaesthetists worked during the daytime, but it offered little more than an area of clinical observation overseen by the nursing staff.

The DGH had a bespoke ITU, admittedly on the second floor, but staffed by the anaesthetists and specially trained nurses.

Previously elderly patients, who had been seen in the Casualty Department and required admission, had to be transferred by ambulance to an array of different hospitals. The DGH had a 30 bedded Geriatric Ward specifically for elderly patients who had been admitted as emergencies.

The Children's ward in the old hospital was small, with children of all ages from babies to teenagers being lumped together.

The DGH had two children's wards, where the segregation of children by age and sex was possible, and with outside courtyards as play areas provided for convalescent children.

However, the DGH's functional deficiencies played a major part in the hospital becoming dysfunctional, and the Paediatricians were quick to realise that their new department had a serious omission in so far as the Special Care Baby Unit (SCBU) remained at the Maternity Home some three miles away on the other side of town.

At the DGH there were too few medical and surgical beds to accommodate emergencies, and with elderly emergencies overflowing virtually every day into the surgical wards, routine admissions from the surgical waiting lists often had to be cancelled.

This lack of medical and surgical beds meant that only Black Notley's medical and surgical wards could be closed, whilst the rest of that hospital remained open.

This shortfall in medical and surgical beds in Colchester was made good (temporarily) by converting some redundant psychiatric wards at Severalls Hospital to accommodate more medical and surgical patients.

However this refurbishment was minimal to say the least, and when one of those wards (Jenner Ward) was deemed in need of rewiring in order to satisfy building regulations, the budgeted spend had been pared down to the bare minimum.

The managers in the works department had no concept of the primitive facilities currently available to patients, and appeared to know nothing about medical or nursing practice.

As luck would have it, one of the senior managers from the works department was admitted under my care as a medical emergency.

Rather unprofessionally I prolonged his hospital stay unnecessarily in the hope that his exposure to this blot on the landscape would motivate him to sanction a proper refurbishment and not just simple 'rewiring'.

It worked!

In subsequent years I had toyed with the idea of getting Mrs Thatcher admitted to one of the worst wards on our patch, in order to get her to see sense, but as they say, 'you can take a horse to water, but you can't make it drink', and Mrs Thatcher, even in her own words, 'was not for turning' or taking a drink from a pauper!

As far as hospital closures were concerned, only Myland Hospital was vacated, with inpatient ophthalmic services being transferred to ECH, and the infectious diseases and respiratory medicine beds, being transferred to a refurbished psychiatric ward at Severalls Hospital.

On paper it might have looked as though we had lost no inpatient beds in this fragmentation exercise, with four medical and surgical wards at Black Notley and four smaller medical and surgical wards from ECH being relocated to five medical and surgical wards at the DGH, and four smaller wards on the Severalls Hospital site.

However, these calculations had overlooked the training requirements for junior doctors at Severalls Hospital.

A RCP inspection a few years later, deemed the Severalls Hospital site to be unsuitable for the training of PRHOs, and as a result two of the wards were closed and their medical patients and PRHOs were transferred to the DGH, without any increase in bed capacity being made at the DGH.

Now medical beds really were being lost, while the house building programme in and around Colchester gathered pace and increased the population which the hospital was supposed to serve.

There was an additional handicap which nobody seemed to have spotted whilst the plans for the DGH were being finalised.

The new hospital had no space allocated for the biochemistry, microbiology and histopathology departments.

How on earth were we supposed to operate an acute hospital dealing with emergencies without these services on site?

The solution offered by the 'planners' (fabricators), was to relocate biochemistry and histopathology to a refurbished villa on the Severalls Hospital site, about one mile distant from the DGH, and microbiology to a defunct Public Health laboratory building, which was situated a few hundred yards down Turner Road!

The latter was then found to have a serious problem with subsidence, and had to undergo a £1,000,000 underpinning procedure to make it safe!

Once this bit of inbuilt inefficiency had been grudgingly accepted by the biochemists, histopathologists and microbiologists, there was a comforting realisation amongst their staff that their separation from the hurly burly of the DGH gave them a much more pleasant and peaceful working

111

environment. Their new surroundings grew on them, and they became loathe to go elsewhere!

Coping without immediate access to biochemistry on the DGH site, was a challenge to the rapid processing of emergencies. However, there was a new emerging solution waiting in the wings – Near Patient Testing.

The bespoke ITU was something which the previous hospital service had lacked, and now gave a much better prospect to patients for survival from life threatening conditions. However, since the problem for the majority of these patients was respiratory in nature, it became imperative to have rapid blood gas analysis at hand. Furthermore, the equipment also measured plasma potassium – a key bit of information for the critically sick patient.

Sending samples up the road, and then having to wait more than an hour (sometimes as long as four hours) for a result, was totally unacceptable.

So a blood gas testing apparatus was installed, and the ITU nurses were trained to operate it.

This rankled the biochemists, who felt that their territory had been encroached upon by people who lacked the rigour of the accredited laboratory technician, but at the same time they could not afford to have one technician seconded to the ITU 24/7 unless management was prepared to fund it, and management had absolutely no intention of increasing the biochemistry budget!

This arrangement also benefitted the medical junior staff, who often needed an assessment of blood gasses and potassium on patients in A&E. This annoyed the Anaesthetists whose budget funded this extra activity, because the machine's consumables were quite expensive.

This interdepartmental budgeting tension was indicative of the way in which any attempt to give an holistic approach to patient care was compromised, by the rigid adherence to the growing NHS compartmentalized fiscal ideology.

The next piece of this fantasy jigsaw was to close Black Notley Hospital and the Colchester Maternity Hospital, and transfer these services along with the gynaecology beds from St Mary's Hospital to a new building (the Constable Wing) situated to the west of and completely separated from the DGH.

The Geriatric patients from Black Notley Hospital were then transferred to the two empty medical wards on the Severalls Hospital site.

The Rheumatology and Rehabilitation beds at Black Hospital were closed and not replaced elsewhere, although an enhanced Physiotherapy & Rehabilitation Department was built at St Mary's Hospital, but it lacked the pool, which had made the service at Black Notley so special.

The acute Orthopaedic beds (1 ward) at the DGH were transferred to the Constable Wing and the remaining medical (respiratory medicine and infectious diseases) beds relocated from Severalls Hospital to the vacated acute Orthopaedic ward on the DGH site.

The foundations of the new Constable Wing were about two metres lower than the foundations of the DGH (the result of the sloping terrain), but no proper physical connection had been planned between the two buildings!
Once again the provision of a joined up service had not been uppermost in the planners' minds!

At about this time the Geriatric Office was relocated from St Mary's Hospital to a two story prefab erected just beyond the goods entrance to the hospital. It included outpatient facilities and physiotherapy. Additionally a prefabricated ward was erected in a space close to the mortuary. It was intended predominantly to take geriatric patients which were hampering surgical activity, but became just another medical ward – Great Bentley Ward.

One of the other deficiencies, on the new Turner Road site, was the absence of a Postgraduate Medical Centre (PGMC).

A number of years earlier the medical staff at ECH and several GPs had put up the money to build a PGMC on some vacant ground at the back of ECH. It comprised a library, lecture theatre, and a bar which also served meals at lunchtime. It was a popular venue for medical staff to meet for lunch and a beer whilst exchanging information about their daily life. It also hosted evening postgraduate meetings for staff and GPs, and served as a convenient location for divisional and managerial staff meetings.

The hospital underwrote the running costs, although the profits from the bar also contributed something towards this additional 'drain on patient services'.

The original design had intended the building to be constructed in such a way that it could in the future be dismantled and reassembled on any future site, but the practicality of this design theory was lost in translation to the final edifice.

Once the DGH was opened the PGMC at ECH became redundant as regards a suitable location for lunch, and the profits of the bar dwindled. Being three miles distant from the DGH its library became underused, and it was also less popular for postgraduate purposes.

The medical staff at the DGH urged management to replace this service on the new hospital site, but it took several years of wrangling to achieve our aims, and at the expense of the building – a refurbished villa from the erstwhile Turner Village Hospital – becoming the property of hospital management and therefore open to all members of staff, and a *pied a terre* for the medical staffing offices.

The ownership of the PGMC at ECH was also transferred to hospital management.

Losing the hegemony over this facility became another way in which management wrested power away from medical staff.

The Postgraduate Medical Federation in London, which had responsibilities for the provision of medical library services in the regions' hospitals, was also side-lined.

The penultimate phase of this chaotic centralisation project was to erect yet another standalone building (Gainsborough Wing) at the north end of the DGH site.

On the ground floor it would contain a dedicated Rheumatology Department (but without inpatient beds), a state of the art Rehabilitation and Physiotherapy Department, and a small Geriatric outpatient assessment unit.

The two floors above would provide wards for all the geriatric patients still scattered around the district, and a ward for the

114

beleaguered Chest Physicians, whose patients had in the interim been moved yet again to part of one of the orthopaedic wards in the Constable Wing.

Once the construction of Gainsborough Wing had been completed, there were financial reasons why it could not be opened immediately, and instead it languished as its various parts were slowly commissioned.

The Gainsborough Wing, just like the Constable Wing, was completely and physically separated from the DGH, but on this occasion the ground floor was about two metres higher. There had been the opportunity to build it at the same level as the DGH, but that additional groundwork would have added an estimated £100,000 to the overall cost, and so it was omitted!

Initially there wasn't even a covered walkway between the DGH and the Gainsborough Wing, and that made the movement of patients to and from the DGH a miserable experience for all involved.

Having botched the DGH site, and added two buildings named after famous Suffolk artists namely Constable and Gainsborough, maybe these buildings should have been named after famous (or infamous) Essex artists, starting with, Keating – the notorious art faker!

At last, St Mary's Hospital and the medical beds at Severalls Hospital could be closed.

The neurophysiological service (EEG) and Electromyography service (EMG) were moved into a prefab that had been put up near the Constable Wing, but the Biochemistry and Histopathology labs remained on the Severalls site!

Furthermore ECH still provided the district's Radiotherapy and Cancer service, as well as Ophthalmology, ENT, Dermatology and medical photography/illustration.

Backlog maintenance of the ECH site now required millions of pounds to make good!

Who on earth, in the corridors of power, thought that this represented joined up thinking and forward planning?

16

Rationalisation and Target Setting

During the first few years of the NHS, the hospital complement of beds fell as many of the smaller, less well constructed hospitals were closed. However, there was still a need to reduce 'unnecessary' or extravagant hospital activity.
There were three ways in which these goals were addressed.

1. Promoting **domiciliary visits** by consultants in order to reduce hospital admissions and outpatient activity.

2. Developing **day surgery** facilities, where patients requiring minor surgical procedures could be admitted and discharged on the same day.

3. Accelerating the throughput of patients by setting **targets**.

Domiciliary Visits
In the beginning there was no obvious shortage of acute inpatient beds, but in order to mitigate any future operational pressures, a system whereby hospital Consultants could perform Domiciliary Visits (DVs) at the behest of a GP, was introduced.
The theory was that this measure would reduce the need for admission to hospital or attendance at an outpatient clinic.
This became an extra source of income for the Hospital Consultant, and inevitably was open to abuse.
However, used appropriately, seeing patients in their own home environment did give the Consultant a much clearer insight into

the relevance of the patient's symptoms and physical signs, which might not otherwise be revealed during a typical outpatient appointment.

It was originally intended that the referring GP should be present at the DV, but only once, in my experience did that actually happen.

It was during my Tuesday afternoon's outpatient clinic at the Clacton Community Hospital that I received a request for a DV from Dr Conrad Hewitt. I hadn't met him before, but his reputation, tarnished by a younger more modern tranche of GPs, preceded him. Now at the age of 80 he was still practising medicine in the environs of Frinton, and still had a small but faithful flock of patients registered at his single-handed practice.

By the time I had reached the patient's house, it was already dark.

An old Bentley had been parked nearby.

On dismounting, I was greeted by the driver of the Bentley – a buxom well-endowed middle-aged woman, whom I soon discovered was Dr Hewitt's receptionist and general factotum.

She helped Dr Hewitt out of the car and introduced us.

He was tall, well dressed, walked slowly and had a noticeable stoop.

It was also apparent that the doctor was very hard of hearing and not a little disabled by poor vision.

His receptionist rang the front door bell, and we were ushered up the stairs to the bedroom, where an elderly gentleman was lying semi-recumbent in bed.

In the dim light of a single light bulb suspended from the ceiling, the patient appeared blue-grey and was taking frequent short gasps of breath.

Examination of the chest confirmed the presence of consolidation of the lower left lung associated with a small effusion.

The diagnosis of pneumonia was irrefutable.

Dr Hewitt had already come to the same conclusion, which made the reason for my presence difficult to comprehend, but when I mentioned my intention to admit the patient to hospital, it became clear that it was the patient's fear of hospitals that was the stumbling block because, like many of his generation, he believed that a hospital was where you were sent to die!

Earlier that day a drug representative had given me a free sample of Amoxil.

I fished it out of my bag, advising the patient's wife to administer one capsule three times daily, and for Dr Hewitt to fill out a new prescription on the following day if the patient's condition appeared to be improving. Otherwise hospital admission would be mandatory.

Pre-empting that event, Dr Hewitt's dutiful receptionist had already filled out an FP10 form, and offered it to Dr Hewitt for his signature.

Since everything had happened so quickly, I came to realise that this was how things were done in Dr Hewitt's practice.

The patient was relieved, the patient's wife was contented, and Dr Hewitt seemed to be happy, although in view of his deafness, I wasn't sure.

Two days later I phoned Dr Hewitt's surgery.

His receptionist answered and told me that the patient had made a miraculous recovery, and his wife had been volubly grateful for the magic pills which I had taken out of my bag!

A few months after that visit, I heard that the Local GP Management Committee (LMC) had advised the GMC to revoke Dr Hewitt's licence to practice on the grounds of him being unsafe.

Dr Hewitt's *raison d'être* had been the practice of medicine.

That had been his life.

Without the practise of medicine, he might as well be dead.

He died six months later!

Seeing a patient in their home environment usually adds a clinical dimension otherwise denied to the Hospital Consultant.

Questions, like asking the patient about their alcohol consumption, are difficult to interpret and commonly misleading, but seeing the empty gin bottles outside a patient's back door was on one occasion far more informative.

Sometimes the DV provided information usually unobtainable in the outpatient scenario – for example, the fortuitous diagnosis of profound myxoedema affecting the patient's wife; and the discovery of a toxic chemical causing a patient's illness.

After being in place for several decades DVs were phased out, usually at the behest of hospital management committees or PCTs on account of it being an uncontrollable cost pressure.

In 2018, The National Institute for Health & Clinical Excellence (NICE) published an assessment of the value of the DV. In spite of a vast number of references, NICE concluded that it was unable to justify the value of the DV in the medical management of patients in the community!

Day Surgery

A day surgery unit requires the use of capital to construct the necessary infrastructure and equip it appropriately.

The Colchester Surgeons had no difficulty persuading the Hospital Board to buy into this new venture.

The unit had two operating theatres and an endoscopy suite.

This was christened the Elmstead Day Centre.

The pre-operative and post-operative accommodation for the patients was primitive and more like a unisex Nightingale Ward, with trolleys instead of beds, but it worked well and patients were not ungrateful.

The nursing staff enjoyed the team spirit, and the fact that it did not involve night duty or weekend working. However, unless the hospital employed more medical and nursing staff, it could not make inroads into the surgical waiting lists!

The appointment of more surgeons might reduce the private activity of those already in post, and that became a limiting factor. Nonetheless management saw this venture as another rationale for the reduction of inpatient beds,

Target Setting & Waiting Lists

Even before the inception of the NHS, the capacity of the hospital service do deliver prompt treatment was limited. Patients who were considered to have non-urgent conditions might have to wait for months before they were seen and treated, but life threatening conditions were usually seen promptly.

Allowing waiting lists to grow is akin to allowing inadequately maintained public toilets to cause sewage backup and eventual overflow. Failing to identify and remedy a toilet which is partially blocked will, sooner or later, result in that toilet becoming permanently blocked. Then excessive pressure on the remaining facility is likely to lead to failure of the entire service.

If the doctors and nurses working in A&E are not given the facilities and extra staff to minimise waiting times, then patients back up and begin to block the service.

In 2000, the Minister of Health, reacting to some adverse publicity, introduced 'waiting time targets', believing that prompt treatment could be achieved by greater efficiency alone. However, he failed to realise that achieving faster throughput could not be delivered without giving hospitals more money and more appropriately trained staff.

Targets, for reducing the time from referral to being seen and/or treated, challenged management to find the wherewithal to deliver best practice. The Government used targets to penalise the service where these arbitrary targets were not met. This also challenged the honesty of consultants not to manipulate long waiting times as a means of increasing their remuneration from Private Practice.

In regard to efficiency and productivity, in 2003 the CEO at our DGH asked our Medical Director (MD), an ENT surgeon, to audit the time taken by different surgeons to perform similar operative procedures. Surgeons resented being required to document the starting and finishing times for every operation. This made the MD exceedingly unpopular.

The limited results obtained were very difficult to assess for the simple reason that some surgeons were more meticulous, had more complicated patients to operate upon, or naturally operated more slowly. Encouraging a surgeon to operate more quickly could lead to errors and unacceptable mistakes, such as severing the ureter during a routine hysterectomy.

When I was a surgical PRHO, one of the surgeons whom I 'assisted' in the operating theatre would ligate or cauterise every bleeding point as soon as they arose, whereas the other surgeon waited until he could no longer see what he was doing before dealing with bleeding points. The latter completed most surgical procedures quite quickly, but his patients suffered from many serious post-operative complications.

With regard to patients referred as emergencies, in the early years of the NHS, these either presented themselves to the Casualty (A&E) Department, or were referred directly to hospital by their GPs.

GP referrals were usually made on the assumption that the patient would be admitted, and thus the patient went directly to the ward of the team 'on call' for the day. However, many of these patients required little more than sorting out their pre-existing medical condition and then returning them to the community. Therefore the temporary occupancy of a hospital bed was neither in the best interests of the patient nor the efficient running of the hospital. Furthermore, particularly at night, the toing and froing of the patient, especially for a radiological examination, caused disruption to the settled ward environment.

The immediate solution was to have all GP referrals start their hospital journey in A&E, and only be admitted to a ward when this early assessment had been completed.

In Colchester the A&E Consultant took exception to this practice and demanded a Casualty Ward where some A&E attenders could be admitted for observation pending their discharge or planned admission, but he would have to wait until the DoH sponsored the development of Medical Assessment Units (MAUs) before that wish was granted.

The MAU
In Colchester this first involved the erection a 'temporary' ward (Great Bentley Ward) to take the patients from the Geriatric Ward (Mersea Ward), and the refurbishment of the Geriatric Ward plus a small part of the contiguous Paediatric Ward to form a MAU.

A £1m government handout was squeezed into just five days of frenetic planning activity. The upshot was that barely half of the money earmarked for the project was spent on the MAU, while the remainder went into the bottomless pocket of the finance department.

Short-changing this new department was a grave error!

When the Labour Government introduced the four hour waiting time target of 98% for patients seen in A&E Departments, they failed to see that this might become an impediment to the way in which A&E patients were assessed in order to ensure that the sickest patients always took priority, and the waiting time for less urgent patients could be legitimately prolonged. It also inferred that some patients waited for excessively long periods because the doctors and nurses were relaxing drinking coffee, or were just lazy!

There were patients who bowled up to A&E with trivial problems which they could have sorted out by themselves.

They seemed to have forgotten that treatment by the NHS was not a <u>right</u> but a <u>privilege</u>, and privileges should not be abused!

MAUs very conveniently helped struggling hospitals to meet the 98% four hour waiting time target, by receiving patients which challenged to breach that goal. Where this wasn't sufficient to assist the hospital meeting that four hour wait, other devious strategies were employed such as making patients who had arrived in ambulances, wait outside the A&E Department, or delaying the registering of new arrivals.

Targets should not have been used to punish the workforce, but as a carrot for management to facilitate efficiency as well as spending more money on infrastructure and staffing.
The only place for target setting is to force managers to increase capacity and/or the staffing at the pinch points in the patient's hospital journey, and if that is financially impossible, then the DoH should shell out more money.

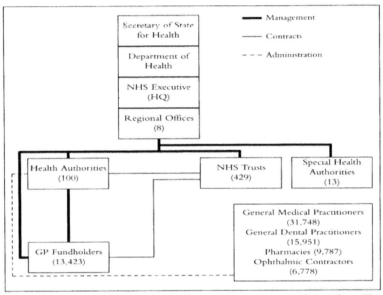

Source: Department of Health, *Departmental Report,* Cm. 3612 (London: The Stationery Office, 1997), annex E.

English Healthcare Administration 1997

PART V

Dismembering the NHS Carcase

17

Management Takeover

Whilst those tasked with delivering healthcare at the coalface were side-lined by engaging in professional elitism, the managers were busy wresting control from the healthcare professionals. The more athletic manipulators were scrambling over each other to climb to the top of the various pyramids, artificial hierarchies and quangos, which had little concern about the welfare of patients.

In this saga the politicians were aided and abetted by the age old method of 'Divide and Rule', with the two major medical combatants being the Hospital Consultants and the GPs.

The interests of Consultants were guarded by the Hospital Consultants & Specialists Association (HCSA), founded in 1948.

The interests of GPs were guarded by the BMA, founded in 1856.

Doctors by and large were too busy empire building to realise that their control over medical decision making would in future be decided by political manoeuvring, both from inside and outside the profession.

In 1975, when I started my life as a Hospital Consultant, there was a well-organised medical managerial system in place.

Hospital medical strategy and decision making were part of what was known as the 'Cogwheel' system.

The medical and surgical Consultants were separated into subcommittees or 'Divisions', which shared the same specialty interests, namely Medical, Surgical or Psychiatric.

It wasn't long before these were subdivided, e.g. the Medical Division spawned the Paediatric and Geriatric Divisions.

As the latest recruit to the hospital, I soon found myself being given the arduous task of 'Medical Division Secretary'. Nobody wanted this job, so it was always imposed upon the latest recruit.

The job involved organising the agenda and taking minutes of each meeting, which came round all too frequently. The minutes went to a central depository and were shared with the other divisions.

The only advantage of this onerous job was that after two years the Secretary automatically became the next Divisional Chairman, unless there were serious objections voiced by the other committee members.

Divisional Chairmen all came together at regular Medical Executive Committee (MEC) meetings, where the divisional minutes were presented and, when relevant, discussed.

One of the most important functions of this committee was to make decisions about the purchase of equipment and agree on enhancements to medical staffing.

The MEC Chairman would then take our wishes to the Hospital Management Committee, which had representatives from all the other parts that make up the hospital environment, and especially the nurses.

There was another committee, to which all medical staff belonged – the MAC.

This committee elected its own Chairman and it was his task to oversee fair play, particularly when there might be grievances from members who might have felt that they had been short-changed by the management hierarchy.

The MAC also vetted applicants for new Consultant posts, and convened a pre-interview sherry party for those who had been short-listed, so that our representative at the finite Regional Board interview could explain our recommendations.

All in all there was a lot of non-medical work that one could get embroiled with if one had the stomach and time to devote to these honorary functions.

Most of us tended to avoid them like the plague, unless we had a very specific point to make, and that attitude, rather than trying to simplify the system, would be our eventual downfall, when professional managers took over the running of the whole healthcare scenario in general, and our local hospitals in particular.

This denouement started in 1984 when DGHs became Hospital Trusts, abolishing the Cogwheel system of medical representation, and replacing it by a set of Directorates. Thereafter each Directorate had their 'own' budget and a Divisional Medical Director appointed by the Board, and not by the medical staff which he represented. It then became the task of these management appointees, who received a generous financial reward for their services, to pass on the immutable decisions made by management.

The MAC remained as before, but its Chairman had no place on the Hospital Board.

At that time the current Chairman of our Medical Division, AHEM, just stepped over the threshold into the new system, without our members playing any part in that takeover.

Members of what was left of the erstwhile Medical Division, could in theory meet with their representative at his meetings with the various non-medical parts of the Medical Directorate, but we also chose to continue to meet from time to time as the 'Physicians Council', where we would discuss whatever we thought was of importance, even though we had no official means of providing the necessary leverage to change the practice of medicine!

However, in 1996, when we discovered that AHEM had failed to inform us, until it was too late for us to submit a business case, of a capital 'grant' of about £1m, which we could bid for to enhance our services, we chose to impeach him and force him to resign his post on the Hospital Board. The Board were unhappy with our action, but could not force our Director to remain on the Board.

Thereafter we were invited to submit applications for the vacant post. Sadly for us, the applicant chosen by the Board, DSHEM, was a politically manipulative Consultant who quickly persuaded the Board to approve the appointment of two additional senior members to his speciality, despite the Physician's Council having been pressing for the appointment of another Consultant Physician, in order to ameliorate the 'on call' burden of emergency care.

As doctors I think we find it difficult to forego a personal departmental enhancement in favour of the greater good, but perhaps we are no different from other people in public office.

The DSHEM and his staff did not contribute to 'on call' emergency medical care!

18

Continuing Professional Development

Political interference was not limited to our day to day clinical activities, it also became a factor in post graduate medical education.

When I was appointed as Consultant Physician with a 'special interest in Endocrinology', the vast majority of doctors, who had achieved their goals of becoming a GP or a hospital Consultant, continued to keep abreast of medical developments by reading the two most popular medical publications – the BMJ and Lancet.

For a tiny minority of doctors, their knowledge base remained fixed at the level they had achieved when they began their definitive appointments. This did not necessarily mean that they were either incompetent or a hazard to patients, because they usually knew where to refer patients whose medical problems were beyond their own limited capabilities.

At the inception of the NHS each district hospital sent representatives from the various specialties to the NETMRB's own Advisory Committees, and the Chairmen from each specialty Committee met at the Regional Board in a two way exchange of ideas to discuss policy and reaction to new governmental dictats.

Within the North East Thames Region, the Endocrinology Advisory Committee did not include members from our region's teaching hospitals, because the teaching hospitals were part of a different NHS management and funding structure.

In a subsequent NHS reorganisation, the specialty committee structure was abolished, but in a move to preserve our potential voice in future NHS developments, our Endocrine Section rebranded itself as the North East Thames Region Association of Clinical Endocrinologists (NETRACE). The officers (Chairman and Secretary) remained the same, and the representatives from our region's 13 district hospitals continued to be its members, but meetings became erratic and unstructured.

In due course we invited representatives from our teaching hospitals to take part in this change of ideas, but they were either too busy or just reluctant to attend our meetings.

One of the ways in which we kept members of NETRACE involved was by getting a pharmaceutical company to sponsor *ad hoc* meetings on occasional Wednesday evenings.

A central location in London was chosen (an upstairs room over a public house) where an evening meal was provided by the landlord, and projection equipment was provided by the drug company representative.

These were pleasant, homely and usually educationally instructive, with one or more members giving a clinical presentation, although for me organising each meeting and the making of the hour-long journey from Colchester to London was rather time consuming.

Then in the early 1990s Professor Kenneth Calman, a well-respected Clinical Oncologist, was invited to chair a committee tasked with the modernisation of medical training. This was a political initiative designed to improve patient safety by ensuring that future Consultants would have appropriately structured and supervised postgraduate training.

The recommendations of this committee were published in 1993 and involved, amongst other considerations, the abolition of the Registrar grade and the creation of the Specialist Registrar Grade (SpR). Most registrars could choose the specialty into which they wished to be absorbed, but numbers of each speciality in the various regions were limited. However, since every NHS Region had their own quotas, candidates could also choose the Region in which to enrol.

It also meant that less popular specialities, such as Geriatrics, were filled by the less fortunate Registrars.

Both the Registrar and Senior Registrar grades were in this way abolished, but many Registrars fell by the wayside or became supernumerary SHOs, and the SHO grade became the new bottleneck in the postgraduate doctor's educational journey.

The Medical Royal Colleges provided the SpR training programmes and peopled the committees to oversee 'fair play'.

In the NE Thames Region this innovation effectively removed the voice of NETRACE, although our members were able to attend the training programme meetings, and were welcomed at Specialist Training lectures, almost exclusively held in the various London teaching hospitals. This added an extra source of continued education for those who had already been appointed with a 'special interest in' as 'Specialty Consultants' in the sticks, and wished to avail themselves of the service.

The downside of this denouement was that DGHs required those accredited in General Medicine to provide the cover for emergency admissions and many hospitals were too small to appoint someone with a single highly specialised specialty accreditation.

In my case, most of my work was involved in general medical activities, but with a single outpatient clinic for specialist endocrinology referrals and another clinic for patients with diabetes.

Whereas previously keeping abreast of changes in medical practice had been voluntary, in the 1980s the DoH and the politically minded doctors amongst our ranks made postgraduate education mandatory, under the umbrella of 'Continued Professional Development' (CPD).

Thereafter doctors had to provide evidence of their postgraduate activity and complete a specific number of hours of approved postgraduate education every year. The politicians saw this as a means of reducing the level of litigation based on 'incompetence' or 'neglect'. A cynic might say that it also gave our professional bodies another way to earn money!

This might have been acceptable if it had subsequently been subjected to audit, but like most dictats, proof of effectiveness was rarely part of any new directive. Instead it just became added to the bureaucratic fog that increasingly enveloped the medical profession.

It would have been far more sensible just to warn doctors that, in the event of litigation for 'incompetence' or 'neglect', they should show evidence of having partaken in postgraduate studies and that would have mitigated against being labelled as an 'ignorant dinosaur'.

Deciding what counted as CPD was a bit arbitrary.

In my first PRHO appointment my boss, Dr Lister, ran a regular lunchtime journal club meeting at Windsor's King Edward VII Hospital, to which he expected his Medical Registrars from the two other hospitals, where he had beds, to attend.

My Registrar took me along to a couple of these meetings.

The Registrars were tasked with the responsibility of reading certain medical journals, such as the BMJ, Lancet, and New England Journal of Medicine, and were then expected to present and discuss articles of interest. This educational menu was helped down with coffee and sandwiches provided by the catering department.

I must say that I was very impressed and, when I was appointed as a hospital Consultant, I set up a similar journal club meeting for the further education of our junior doctors, and a variety of pharmaceutical company representatives willingly provided the sponsorship that paid for the lunch.

Everybody got something out of these meetings and it cost management nothing, but in the fullness of time, when management were asked to underwrite the expense of running our postgraduate centre, they began to become rather less than helpful!

In Colchester our Journal Club was Consultant lead, and was intended more for the further education of the junior staff rather than the Consultants, but attending these meetings counted towards our annual requirement of CPD.

In 1986, medical Audit became a compulsory part of every hospital doctors' contract. As far as management was concerned, this would serve more as a means of focussing doctors' minds on the cost of delivering healthcare, rather than improving outcomes.

In Colchester one of the surgeons was appointed to galvanise this new activity and by default I became the organiser of audit for the Physicians and our related non-surgical specialties. £15,000 was made available for the purchase of hardware and software to facilitate this activity, and unsurprisingly the Surgeons took the lion's share of this handout.

The Physicians began by holding their audit meetings in one of the DGH's pokey little meeting rooms on every Friday morning before the day's clinical work was due to begin.

The initial theme was to look at inpatient deaths which had been selected by the medical records department, and at each meeting two or three cases, admitted under one of the Consultants' teams, would be chosen for discussion.

It was my task to make a record of each meeting, and then send a report to the audit office.

Criticising patient management by your colleagues inevitably became muted for fear of 'payback' when it was your own turn to sit on the hot seat.

Audit became seen as divisive and counterproductive. Consequently this death audit was changed to case presentations, which encouraged a theatre for one-upmanship!

When the new hospital finally acquired a PGMC, it was chosen as the venue for these meetings, which became much more elaborate clinical case presentations with contributions from other specialties. They also encouraged drug companies to fund the provision of coffee and some solid nourishment, for those who had not had time to take breakfast.

Somehow the medics had taken back the initiative, and ignored the effect that audit might have to reduce hospital expenditure!

Attending these Friday morning clinical presentations, also counted towards our annual CPD requirements, but these in-house activities were by themselves not enough to satisfy the authorities, and therefore attending educational meetings outside one's locality was also required.

The scope for educational self-betterment had been there long before CPD became compulsory.

The medical and surgical colleges had extensive libraries and regularly sponsored postgraduate meetings, which in turn provided their college with additional income.

For those of us who retained a keen interest in the science which underpinned the art of medical practice, there were national and international meetings to attend, giving us a breather from the day to day delivery of healthcare. We could pick and choose which meetings would be most interesting and then rearrange our clinical duties so that we still fulfilled our contractual obligations. Unfortunately the latter was not always possible and so we missed out on many of those particular opportunities.

Royal Society of Medicine (RSM) held a smorgasbord of educational activities in London with annual one day specialty meetings around the country.

In order to avail ourselves of these facilities, there was a very generous study leave allowance with most expenses paid, although travel abroad was only reimbursed if we were presenting a paper or participating in some other way at a conference.

On some occasions a drug company sponsored our expenses.

These away-days were a pleasure and not a chore.

GPs, who were in effect self-employed, could only claim such meetings as tax allowable expenses, although many of them enjoyed a dubious conflict of interest by accepting sponsorship from pharmaceutical companies. However, this practice was eventually outlawed, except where it could be shown that there had been no overt promotion of any pharmaceutical product.

The GPs held evening meetings at our PGMC at which invited speakers, from the medical staff or from outside the hospital, gave talks on a wide variety of medical topics.

The opportunities for personal CPD were there for the taking.

When the government stepped in to regulate CPD, the paperwork entailed to quantify this function became a real bore, although it did allow one to drop one of one's clinical sessions. Clearly the voluntary nature of personal improvement was lost at the expense of reducing the time devoted to patient care.

Did anyone care about that?

19

Outsourcing Services and PFI

As soon as management had taken the reins from the medical staff, they could drive the healthcare coach wherever their fancy took them, and removing non-medical functions from the balance sheet would have been the natural way in which big business had usually addressed efficiency.

Since staff are the biggest cost pressure, staff reduction/redundancy is the easiest way to save money!

Services such as laundry, cleaning, catering, porterage and security were all areas where savings could be made. This could be either addressed in house or by getting a second party to take over the service. With the second option, the space on the hospital campus, previously occupied by those erstwhile members of staff, could be used for other purposes or simply demolished. The actual savings were likely to be small but, in order for the Private Sector to provide these services and make a profit, standards were likely to be compromised.

Transferring staff to a new service provider was carried out by a process called 'TUPE' (Transfer of Undertakings Protection of Employment). It was intended to guarantee the employee's right to continued employment, but if the takeover exercise was intended to involve a reduction of staffing levels, then since the safeguards were cumbersome, ways around the legislation were used.

In the farming community, being 'tupped' is what happens when a ram has mounted a ewe, i.e. the ewe having been shafted!
Likewise affected members of staff felt that they were being tupped!

141

When catering in Colchester was offered to the Private Sector, a group from our hospital catering staff clubbed together and set up a their own cook-chill service in the defunct Severalls Hospital kitchens. It worked very well even though transporting meals to the various hospitals in our district added an extra cost and thereby reduced the venture's profitability.

Eventually they were superseded by a national consortium operating at a distance but, with a much greater clientele base, they could outbid and undercut our local service.

This was all about big business making a profit and not about giving patients a better choice or quality of food.

However, the outsourcing of non-essential services could not deal with the cost of capital developments, and so the removal of the government's responsibility for providing the capital for building projects and infrastructure maintenance was the next step taken by the Chancellor of the Exchequer to wash his hands of making improvements to the hospital campus.

With Britain a member of the European Economic and Monetary Union (EMU), we were obliged to keep public debt below a certain threshold called the Government debt-to-GDP ratio. The Private Finance Initiative (PFI) was seen as a mechanism to take debt off the government balance sheet and thus meet this part of the Maastricht Convergence Criteria.

However there was little active participation in this foible until after the 1997 Parliamentary election.

With a 179-seat majority (33 more seats than Clement Atlee's 1945 record breaking majority), the neocapitalist reign of Tony Blair's New Labour Government began to show their hidden capitalist credentials.

The Labour Minister of Health, Alan Milburn, who had visited the *Universitario Fundación Alcorcón* hospital in Madrid, saw a way around the various punitive NHS funding handicaps.

Apparently the Spanish National Health System had funded the building of that hospital, and then allowed a private company to take on that debt, thereby exempting it from many of the rules normally imposed on state-owned hospitals.

In that way PFI could streamline capital developments and free the hospital from some of central government's red tape. However, opening the NHS to the marketplace included the biggest player in the capitalist world, namely London's faceless moneylenders, and they have no truck with charity. Herein was the Achilles' heel of PFI, because the inflation-proofed 'mortgage' repayments could cripple the ability of the hospital to deliver care, whilst giving the Private Sector a gift wrapped profit, and the NHS a chronic financial headache.

This was another manifestation of the 'Plastic Revolution' of 'have now, pay later', which had become firmly entrenched in the population.

The wise used the system cautiously.

The foolish embraced this spending spree irresponsibly.

Those in the Government, who were legally up to their necks in the usury business, were not bothered about leaving the Treasury in hock to the debt collectors.

All they needed to do was to make sure that the legislation in force protected their interests and blamed the local hospital if it defaulted on its repayments!

For the naïve, PFI now offered an alternative way out of Colchester's hospital infrastructural mess which had accumulated since the inadequately resourced DGH had been opened in 1985.

Our CEO at the time had previously attempted to make our hospital a Foundation Hospital Trust (FHT), which would have given us the means to borrow the money to construct the necessary improvements, but our long surgical waiting list had been cited as something that had to be addressed before a formal application could go ahead.

Consequently about £4 million was spent reducing waiting lists, with the Private Sector providing the beds and operating facilities, whilst our surgeons gladly cashed in on the bonanza. However, instead of persevering with the FHT dream, our CEO adopted the alternative strategy offered by using PFI as the means to enhance our hospital.

143

In 2003 that ball was set in motion, and applicants for the post of Medical Advisor were sought. Since I had just retired, I put my name forward and, after a gruelling interview, became the successful candidate.

Like many recently retired doctors I found it difficult to drop the baton. I had already agreed to do one outpatient session per week, because the Hospital Trust had not appointed my successor. Adding two sessions per week as the PFI Medical Advisor gave me an extra interesting challenge, and I also had an honorary contract which allowed me to complete a research project, which I had been working on for several years.

With the Hospital Trust's Medical Director kindly offering me a *pied-à-terre* in his office, I felt buoyed up.

There followed a number of public meetings to look at our district's healthcare needs, and our local GPs played a significant role in facilitating the venture.

This also coincided with a government sponsored set of meetings between 2003 and 2004, 'The Emergency Services Collaborative', which I attended along with other colleagues from our hospital, including a presentation on the diagnosis and management of Deep Venous Thrombosis (DVT) by one of our senior MAU nurses. The critical word was **Collaboration** and the sharing of best practice, and not about **Competing** for resources.

In Colchester the nurses on our MAU had pioneered a different way of managing patients with a suspected DVT – a common reason for GP referral to hospital. Up until that time these patients would have been admitted for one or more days whilst a diagnosis was established and, when indicated, anticoagulant therapy commenced.

The new scheme involved no inpatient stay.

All the investigations, including outpatient management of anticoagulant therapy, were completed on the day of arrival, saving an average of six inpatient days – a much better experience for patients and a significant reduction in costs, but did management reward staff or the department for this change of practice?

One of the other outcomes of this 'collaborative' was to promote the amalgamation of the A&E and MAU into a single unified point of entity at the front door of the hospital, with the name changing to 'Emergency Department' (ED), rather than A&E. This was an area of healthcare which I felt passionately about, but it did tend to deflect my attention from the other needs of our hospital.

Our local PFI team went to see how the newly constructed Norfolk & Norwich Hospital, built as a PFI, had embraced this concept. Sadly their emergency service had been divided between two separate locations, and on the morning of our visit, their capacious A&E Department was almost empty with the nurses chatting and drinking coffee, whilst their MAU and Surgical Assessment Unit (SAU) were heaving, with the nurses' feet barely touching the ground!

They had also built that hospital with too few beds!

Clearly we did not intend our PFI to have the same design fault!

Our PFI went through all the necessary processes before appointing a preferred provider, and then got on with the business of welding the plans into a coherent project.

Throughout this time the local PCT kept throwing spanners in the works, demanding amongst other things that we reduce the cost of the scheme – something that was almost impossible without losing some of its functionality.

At that time the PCT was involved in a Local Investment Finance Trust (LIFT) project to build a new community health centre, and relocate their offices therein.

This conflict of interest caused several months of delay to the negotiation of our own PFI! Furthermore nobody fully appreciated that one of the reasons for the PFI being so costly, was that we could not give the construction company access to the whole site, and that piecemeal construction had to precede the process of tying all the parts together.

This adds time, and time in the construction industry adds costs!

When we were close to signing off the PFI with our chosen provider, Andy Burnham – the Minister of Health – announced a temporary moratorium on all hospital PFI projects, and advised those involved to find ways of reducing their costs.

We also lost our dynamic CEO, who had just been appointed to a lucrative managerial healthcare role in Jersey.

His replacement, Peter Murphy, came in the form of a hospital manager who had previously been involved in the downgrading of King George Hospital in Ilford, in order to help finance the new Queen's Hospital (PFI) in Romford.

Not a good omen!

Had he been a willing facilitator in the destruction of **his** local hospital, or did he find himself under the thumb of his political masters?

We had not chosen him.

Did he have the talents and the authority to relieve Colchester of our dysfunctional hospital?

Within a few months it was clear that our new CEO was looking at ways of cancelling our PFI on the grounds that the repayment schedule would be unaffordable.

In the summer of 2006, our PFI team was given 24 hours to come up with a cost saving plan.

We spent the day in one of the conference rooms of the nurse training school on the Severalls Hospital site, trying our hardest to come up with a solution. One of our suggestions was the conversion of one of the new wards to a private patient ward. This was something which we estimated would provide the hospital with an additional annual return of about £1 million.

However, even that was not deemed sufficient to make the PFI affordable, and the plug was duly pulled!

Most of the members of the PFI team already had jobs in the hospital, so they would not lose out. Losing my remuneration was of little consequence because I already had my NHS pension. However, the project director, the project manager and a few other employees would be out of a job.

Rather cleverly, the CEO offered the director and manager well paid jobs within the Trust!

With that fall-back position, were they likely to oppose the abandonment of the PFI?

Hardly!

Penalty clauses in the original engagement contract cost the taxpayer an estimated £10 million.

At a public meeting a few months later, our CEO explained that it would be better for the Trust's finances for it to become a Foundation Hospital Trust (FHT), because that would give us a more sustainable way of funding a similar building project.

His predecessor had been there before, but had not attempted to use all the devious financial ways in which the hurdles could be jumped successfully.

Nobody acknowledged the fact that some project directors in the Midlands and north of England had found innovative ways of mitigating the impact of an otherwise unaffordable PFI.

However, this was not so in Colchester, and an alternative agenda replaced the original plan to build and refurbish a modern well integrated hospital.

The mood at that public meeting had been acrimonious, but the surgeons were uncharacteristically silent.

Later it became clear that our CEO would have been unable to pull the rabbit out of the hat without the help of the Surgeons.

The reasons for the opposition of the Surgeons to the PFI were twofold, and the pausing of the PFI process by the Health Minister gave them the opportunity to take charge.

Firstly, there was the Elmstead Day Surgery Unit.

This was a sort of sacred cow for the Surgeons, who had fought hard to get it built, and the PFI would have demolished it and incorporated the day surgery operating theatres into a new operating theatre complex in the main hospital.

The nurses from the day surgery unit feared that their special status would be removed, and they would have to take part in the main hospital theatre staff duty rosters.

Nurses working in the day unit neither had to work at night nor at weekends – a privilege which they were loath to give up.

Secondly, the Vascular Surgeons had been planning to make Colchester a centre for major abdominal vascular surgery, and by so doing poach patients from Ipswich Hospital. This would have been a lucrative venture, but with a PFI crippling the hospital's finances, there would not have been the capital resources available to equip an appropriate operating theatre.

So with the Surgeons in the CEO's pocket, or the CEO in the Surgeons' pocket, there was nothing that anyone else could do about this *volte face*.

Sometimes there is a need to subjugate one's personal speciality interests in favour of the greater good – but not in this case!

In regard to our poor emergency services, the medical staff did not hold the purse strings, and were not in the driving seat!

My naïvety had resulted in me letting the hospital down, but at least our CEO did pledge that with FHT status achieved, he would give priority in any future building project, to the construction of a modern ED, and the relocation of Cancer Services along with the other departments still languishing at ECH.

FHT status was achieved a couple of years later, but in the interim, with the assistance of the Medical Directorate Manager (our erstwhile PFI Manager), I had put together a scheme whereby most of the hospital's functional deficiencies could be overcome. The plan involved the erection of a four storey building between the Gainsborough Wing and the main hospital, with Radiotherapy in the basement, an ED on the ground floor and the Pathology Department on the top floor.

In 2009 I showed the plans to our CEO, who was generally supportive provided that he could raise the capital (about half of what the PFI would have cost), and the Director of Nursing gave it her blessing. Then with encouragement from one of the NEDs, a retired nephrologist from Chelmsford, I gave a Power Point presentation to our assembled MAC.

148

However, the Surgeons had not been idle, and by this time they had an 'oven-ready' project to replace the Great Bentley Ward prefab, with a new Paediatric Department and their bespoke surgical ward on the floor above.

Then I queered their pitch by drawing attention to some functional defects in those plans, whereupon the Medical Director, incensed by my interference, revoked my honorary Consultant status, and effectively banned me from the hospital campus.

He had found that I was no longer registered with the GMC, which he erroneously thought had been an essential condition for me to continue to conduct a longstanding research project at the hospital! However, since my role did not involve 'medical practice' his objection was flawed, but what could I do about it?

In order to get my name back on the GMC list, I would have to travel to London for an interview, re-provide the paperwork which the GMC already had, and pay a special additional fee. All in all a timewaster and a waste of money, but long enough for their building project to go ahead without any more objections from me!

A few years later, when this CEO was replaced, none of his original pledges had been honoured, but the Vascular Surgeons had been provided with a brand new building and radiological equipment which would make it possible for Colchester to poach major abdominal vascular surgery from Ipswich Hospital.

I sat next to Peter Murphy our CEO at a Medical Society dinner just before his departure. He came across as a mild mannered man, who had found himself unwillingly saddled with an uncaring political agenda.

He told me that he had recently completed the construction of a patio at the back of his house, despite having never done any DIY before.

He admitted that it was not perfect, but it had given him a sense of achievement, which he had never experienced in his whole career working for the NHS as a manager!

In retrospect, abandoning the PFI had been the right decision, because all over England other PFIs were bankrupting their hospitals and setting the scene for giving NHS hospitals to the Private Sector, or amalgamating failing Hospital Trusts with neighbouring 'more efficient' hospitals, but this did not stop services to patients from deteriorating.

I had obviously not fully realised that in this new healthcare scenario patients did not come first!

20

The Foundation Hospital Trust

The motivation behind the Government's plan to give FHT status to all NHS hospitals is not altogether clear, but political explanations do not necessarily reveal the truth and more commonly are concerned with expediency!

In 1948 when the NHS spacecraft was launched into imaginary space, little detailed thought had been given on how to keep it in orbit.

There were airy fairy notions that as health inequality was reduced, the need for ongoing medical care would also be reduced, and in that way the cost of providing the service would not get out of hand.

Increasing the expectation of life was seen as a blessing.

With more people continuing in work and contributing to the economy until they reached retirement age, the wheels of commerce would be able to afford to keep the NHS solvent in spite of expensive new investigative procedures and treatments. However, with pensioners becoming an increasing proportion of the population, and chronic disease accumulated along the way and dominating their need for medical care, the scales began to become tipped against the survival of the NHS as it had originally been conceived.

It was easy for politicians to turn a blind eye to the size and depth of this iceberg, because the provision of social care had been carefully kept in the remit of the local authorities.

Be that as it may, the shekel shufflers in government soon realised that they would need to come up with wheezes that offloaded the cost of healthcare onto the risk-taking Private Sector, which might not be too concerned about the standard of care, provided that their backers made a profit.

Selling nationally owned and run industries to the Private Sector put money into the Treasury and reduced the cost of running the country.

These were typical Tory values, and the same values that have allowed the Tory tail to wag the British dog to death.

In November 1971, the Secretary of State for the Environment granted outline planning approval for a National Exhibition Centre (NEC) to be built in Birmingham. This would be a project paid for and owned by the Birmingham City Council.

On 16th February 1973, Prime Minister Edward Heath cut a white ribbon to initiate its construction.

The NEC was opened by the Queen on 2nd February 1976.

The City Council then sold the NEC for £307m to the 'Birmingham NEC Group'.

Three years later the Birmingham NEC Group sold it on for about £800m!

They say that 'money doesn't grow on trees', but capitalist family trees are clearly different, and this would be how the Government planned to outsource healthcare and its NHS property portfolio, when most people had forgotten that the NHS real estate had been acquired in the 1948 'fire sale' for next to nothing!

Ever since the inception of the NHS, there had been a lobby of erstwhile healthcare providers, who hankered after a return to the hospital management style which had operated during the first half of the twentieth century. These were people who wanted to be in charge of what was delivered in their locality, without the authoritarian hand of central government dictating the rules, but they had all but forgotten the fact that without the NHS their local hospitals would have been declared bankrupt.

The socialist principle in 1948 was to provide a better standard of hospital care to those areas in Britain, where poverty, unemployment and homelessness had made them hotspots of disease.

Nye Bevan was focussed upon the social deprivation in the Welsh valleys, and he intended to right the wrongs of the capitalist politicians, even if it meant giving less of the national cake to the well-to-do parts of the country.

Almost twenty five years later there seemed to be the opportunity to give local healthcare management back to every part of the country.

From 1974 to 1982 the first attempt at this decentralisation had been the creation of the AHAs, but these just added the cost of providing another layer of bureaucracy, whilst pitting the hospitals in the area against each other in their bid to get more of the cake.

In 1982 AHAs were replaced by District Health Authorities (DHAs).

GP Fundholding was created in 1991 by the Tory Government as part of the quasi-market place, in order to make hospitals compete with each other for GP referrals, but after the Labour Party returned to power in 1997, GP fundholding was scrapped.

New Labour then created 481 PCTs which in effect became the new fund holders and perpetuated the competition between service providers for a share of the market.

Competition between different groups of providers might work in the capitalist world of big business, but it is quite inappropriate in healthcare. What we really needed was cooperation between hospitals and GPs, and sharing the resources in the best way possible for patients.

Throughout the history of NHS reorganisations, the income of the NHS hospital was dependent upon whichever management scenario was in force. It made planning particularly difficult especially when the next year's funding was dependent upon the previous year's performance, and the colour of the political party in charge.

A small proportion of each year's hospital expenditure had been ring-fenced for capital developments, but there was no scope for the transfer of funds between capital development and the cost

153

of delivering the service. Furthermore, if there was any surplus at the end of each financial year, then the unspent money went straight back to the Treasury.

The funding system, which Alan Milburn had seen in Spain, additionally allowed hospitals to negotiate their own contracts with its employees. The only brake on this potential runaway engine was an imposed governance mechanism provided by local government, trade unions, health workers and community groups.

In 2003, the legislation to ape the Spanish model came into force, which allowed the creation of what were described as FHTs, and by 2004 the first ten FHTs had been created.

There was also a new type of service on the block provided by Independent Sector Treatment Centres (ISTCs).

ISTCs were in effect privately owned establishments which specialised in specific treatments such as cataract surgery or joint replacement surgery. They were given five year contracts to deliver a specified number of procedures at prices above the national tariff, and without any financial penalty if the contract had not been fulfilled.

The final seal on this deal came with 'Payment by Results' (PbR) which was a mechanism which enabled healthcare providers to milk the NHS cash cow. PbR consisted of Healthcare Resource Groups (HRGs), which grouped together patient events that had been judged to consume a similar level of resource.

The first national tariffs for 15 HRGs were issued in 2003-04.

The turkey shooting season had begun!

With Colchester's PFI abandoned, every effort was made by management to achieve FHT status.

It may well have been that PFI and the idea of the FHT were conceived simultaneously, but were rolled out at different times. The optimists saw this all singing all dancing establishment on the horizon when in fact all they were seeing was a mirage or pie in the sky, but it took several years for the penny to drop and for that illusion to be shattered.

The reality of the situation was that the FHT was not really concerned with the health of patients, but rather the health of the Treasury.

Historically, the funding mechanism for hospitals progressed in a sequence of legislative initiatives, which started by taking away their financial dependence upon the local community and parking it with the Treasury, and then returning it to a type of local financial independence to feed the FHT.

It sounded quite simple but it was snared in complications which could at the end of the day allow the hospital to be 'bought out' by the Private Sector.

The Board of Management of a FHT was like that of the Hospital Trust which it had replaced and comprised:

> CEO
> Chairman
> Director of Finance
> Director of Human Resources
> Medical Director
> Director of Nursing

To this nucleus other posts could be added, such as a

> Director of Estates
> Director of Operations
> Hospital Secretary

Not all members of the Board had voting rights, and the Chairman could only vote when there was a tie.

A second layer of governance in the form of Non-Executive Directors (NEDs) was added 'in order to keep the Board in check'. They had no voting rights, but were supposed to add a layer of expertise which the Board could call upon in order to complement their activities. Maybe initially it had been hoped that through their influential contacts, the hospital might attract financial investment from big business or Big Pharma.

The NEDs received a small salary for services rendered, and had the power to sack members of the Board. NEDs were also involved in the appointment and dismissal of the CEO and Chairman.

A third layer of governance was added in the form of Governors, who were supposed to call the NEDs to account. They were the unpaid representatives elected by the local community and were misguidedly seen as the guardians of the health interests of the community which they represented.

Governors were elected by the community served by the hospital, but the hospital controlled the mechanism by which Governors were elected. This might not have been seen as a handicap, but as I will show in PART VII, it was a mechanism by which the Board could get away with all sorts of misdemeanours.

Overseeing the competence of the FHT was a quango called Monitor, whose remit was to ensure that the hospital remained financially solvent. Unfortunately therein lay the trap which encouraged the unwary or the foolhardy, who claimed to be able to predict a rosy financial future from an overoptimistic forecast of possible windfalls or unprecedented efficiency savings.

Monitor had little interest in how FHTs delivered healthcare. It was up to the CEO and his Board of Directors to find the ways and means of garnering income from near and far.

Those in charge of the Mid-Staffs Hospital Trust snared themselves in this way during the process of applying to become a FHT (granted in 2007), because within two years of becoming a FHT, Monitor discovered a massive hole in their budget, and a whistle blower revealed the uncaring way in which cuts had resulted in unprecedented patient mortality.

Policing the quality of care delivered by hospitals was addressed in 2003 by the introduction of the Commission for Healthcare Audit and Inspection (CHAI), which was a soft touch, arms-length system which awarded stars according to the quality of care, measured against a number of standards, with the information gathered from patient satisfaction questionnaires and statutory returns from which the Hospital Standardised Mortality Ratio (HMSR) could be calculated.

HMSR was introduced in 1999 and monitored by Imperial College London. It was superseded by the Summary Hospital-level Mortality Indicator (SHMI) in 2011, which included all deaths occurring within 28 days of discharge from hospital, in order to stop hospitals from discharging patients prematurely, in order to give the impression that they had excellent mortality rates.

Had the Mid-Staffs Trust been subjected to greater scrutiny about their excessive death rates from 2005-2008, as part of the process of becoming a FHT, it is unlikely that they would have been given FHT status.

However, death rates are poor indicators of poor nursing care or poor medical practice. The real benchmark should have been 'avoidable' deaths, but this requires a much higher level of scrutiny and a determination to carry out death audits which might expose staff to criticism. Furthermore there was little information available regarding the magnitude of this problem.

In 2009, since CHAI had failed to identify preventable deaths, the Care Quality Commission (CQC) was introduced. It made probing inspections of hospital premises and other parts of the care 'industry', e.g. GP surgeries.

Their inspections were aggressive and could lead to the hospital being put into special measures if the Board had failed to comply with the recommendations of previous inspections, but their inspectors lacked the competence to identify the scale of preventable deaths.

In 2010 this weakness was addressed by the Preventable Incidents Survival and Mortality (PRISM) study.

Dr Hogan, the lead researcher, randomly selected a thousand case notes from the 2009 adult mortality data of ten NHS Trust Hospitals which had agreed to take part in the study. These cases did not include obstetric, psychiatric or palliative care patients or those where there was an ongoing medicolegal inquiry.

A group of retired Consultant Physicians and Surgeons were recruited to examine these case notes and give each a score ranging from 1-6, where 1 represented excellent quality of care and 6 represented very poor care.

Each Consultant volunteer examined 50 case notes. 25% were double checked and all reports, where a preventable cause of death had been identified, were discussed with the lead researcher.

(The results were made public in 2011 and published in the BMJ in 2012 BMJ **2012;21:737–45**.)

157

The research revealed that 5.2% of these hospital deaths had been preventable, and were usually the culmination of a poor or a very poor standard of care, with most cases being multifactorial in nature.
I was one of those volunteers, and it took me over a week to plough through the fifty case notes allotted to me!

Clearly the scale of this problem is huge as well as being unidentified, unless a patient, a patient's friend or relative or a hospital whistle blower makes a complaint.

This problem could be resolved if all hospital deaths were subjected to an independent process of scrutiny, but setting up such a mechanism would be very costly unless the scrutineers were medically trained volunteers, e.g. retired medical practitioners. Clearly FHTs were not going to get involved unless they were forced to comply by legislation.

For the FHT to be financially viable it had to devise ways of appearing to be solvent.

Outsourcing essential activities such as housekeeping, catering, car parking and security had already been addressed.

The outsourcing of nursing had to be less obvious to all but the members of the Board.

There had always been a steady flow of nurses in and out of hospital employment, but previously that had been well balanced in order that very few nursing shortages actually occurred. However, if vacancies were not advertised and only filled temporarily by agency staff, then it was possible to manipulate the nursing establishment to make it look as though the hospital was fully staffed with nurses when in fact there were serious shortages.

Similar wheezes had long been used to cover medical staffing shortfalls, but usually it was possible to get the existing staff to fill those gaps in duty rotas and other clinical functions without shelling out additional salary enhancements.

The main difference between doctors and nurses is that it is the nurses who provide face to face patient care, and when nurse numbers fall below a critical level that personal care to patients suffers.

There is only so much time in a nurse's shift to provide all those things that nurses do so expertly. Of course many nurses were able and willing to go beyond what was demanded of them, but there comes a time when the system breaks under this sort of strain.

Sickness rates among staff increase.
Staffing gaps are not filled.
There is a downward spiral.
Patient care suffers.
Accidents and unexplained deaths increase.
The morale of the staff deteriorates.

Provided that the Board can keep a cap on negative publicity, this process will continue. Even though the staff might know what was going on, they were disinclined to speak out because their future employment depended upon keeping stumm.

In theory FHTs have a failsafe mechanism in the form of their Governors, but the employment contracts of these unpaid public servants made it abundantly clear that their allegiance was to the hospital Board, and not the way in which the Board conducted its business.
That had been the totalitarian approach of the world's dictators!
Was this now the new accepted face of democracy in England?

The Response of Scotland and Wales
The devolved governments of Scotland and Wales were free to develop their own ways of delivering healthcare to their individual populations, and spent the Treasury's money differently.
They did not support the PFI, ISTC or PbR agendas and retained their Area Health Boards instead of going down the PCT or the Clinical Commissioning Group (CCG) pathway, but like England they had to endure the NHS spending cuts.

PART VI

Public Involvement

21

FHT Governors

Prior to the establishment of the NHS, public involvement in healthcare had been mainly concerned with money raising activities in order to maintain the day to day expenditure of the voluntary hospitals, but they also raised the money for specific capital enhancements, e.g. the building of a Children's Ward at ECH.

Additionally, elected members of the public, who sat on local or borough councils, contributed to the agendas of the hospital and community services for which the council was responsible, e.g. the local Fever Hospital.

Hospital Management Committees did not include a public member elected by the local community, although they might appoint a member of the public who shared the committees' objectives, just to give a semblance of public inclusiveness.

With the establishment of FHTs that previous lack of genuine public involvement was addressed by the mandatory inclusion of a Council of Governors elected by the public, but the terms and conditions imposed by the hospital trust could effectively gag these elected members and thereby renderer their contributions useless and mere window dressing.

When the Colchester Hospital Trust was attempting to become a FHT, it first had to encourage the local population to become Members who in turn would be able elect the Governors. At that time public membership was confined to those living in NE Essex, and since I lived just over the Essex Suffolk border, I was not eligible, despite the fact that Colchester's DGH was my local hospital and my GP practice was based in Colchester.

At about the same time the Ipswich Hospital Trust was exploring the possibility of becoming a FHT. It also encouraged the local South Suffolk population to become Members, so that the hospital would be able to hold Governor elections.

In that way I became a Governor of Ipswich Hospital.

Ipswich's Governors' Council met at regular intervals, and I was impressed by the way in which these consultative meetings were conducted by their Chairman.

On several occasions I had a one to one meeting with their CEO, who impressed me with his openness and desire to get suggestions about how the hospital service in Ipswich could be enhanced.

In 2010 Colchester's DGH had been a FHT (CHUFT) for three years and needed to conduct new Governor elections, but on this occasion residents living in South Suffolk were included as well as those from the 'rest' of Essex. This was because one of the conditions imposed on FHTs by the current legislation was that their Membership should represent 1% of their catchment population, or at least the FHT should be seen to making the effort to maintain such a level of membership. Since the hospital provided services to parts of neighbouring South Suffolk and Mid Essex, those areas were then included for recruiting Members.

I put my name up for election and was duly elected.

I was then told by Colchester's Chairperson (SIC) that I could not be a Governor of two FHTs, even though Ipswich had not by that time become a FHT.

The downside of being a Governor at Ipswich was that their meetings were held in the evenings, and returning home by car in the dark was difficult. Furthermore, using public transport to get to Ipswich Hospital involved three different buses and took about 2½ hours. So, although I had been impressed by the attitude of the management at Ipswich Hospital, I chose Colchester, since the car journey of eight miles took less than half an hour, even in heavy traffic.

What I did not realise was that our SIC ruled the Governors with a rod of iron, and had no intention of giving the Governors' Council a free rein.

At the first meeting of this newly formed Governors' Council, we should have elected our Lead Governor, but our SIC decided, without taking a vote, that the previous Lead Governor should continue in that role. This annoyed a handful of the newly elected Governors, who had served during the previous three years. They were not impressed with the leadership of this Lead Governor, especially since he seemed to be in the pocket of our SIC, and would be unlikely to challenge decisions made by the Board.

These 'experienced' Governors told me that the process by which changes to the service were being introduced followed a typical pattern:

The Board develops a plan without consulting the Governors, and then the plan is included in the agenda of the next public meeting of the Governors' Council.

Since hardly any of the Governors had come from a background in healthcare, their ability to understand the details in the paperwork of any new initiative was marginal and, without the opportunity to discuss this initiative in private before the public meeting, they were putty in the hands of any Chairman or CEO.

Subsequently the unaltered plans are given to the press, who are then able to tell the local population that their representatives, the Governors, had given the plans their assent, even though the Governors only role had been to rubber stamp the Board's decisions, but without the prior opportunity to contribute to or examine and question the details.

This farcical fraudulent practice was bound to continue until someone found a way round these obstacles.

In July 2011 I attended a meeting of the Foundation Trust Governors' Association (FTGA) in London. The arrangements were made by Capita, and involved a series of presentations washed down with a lavish lunch.

The FTGA was a side-shoot of Monitor and was concerned with providing 'training' facilities for Governors. FHTs were encouraged to enrol their

Governors at a cost to the hospital of about £3,500 per annum. In this way Governors were enabled to receive the necessary indoctrination in the principles of being the hospital's best 'buddy'. There was also the Foundation Trust Network (FTN), which performed similar functions.
In 2014 the FTGA and the FTN were merged into the Governors Policy Board (GPB) which is now a branch of NHS Providers as defined in the dreadful 2012 Lansley NHS Act of Lunacy.

At the FTGA meeting in 2011, I sat next to a retired professor of clinical chemistry – an international expert on factitious hypoglycaemia. He was totally nonplussed by his own hospital's lack of engagement with their Governors, and the uselessness of this aspect of governance!

In Colchester, during their first three years as a FHT there had been some vague discussions about the promise given by the previous CEO to prioritise the building of a new ED along the lines of our failed PFI, plus the relocation of cancer services from ECH, and ultimately the reprovision of all the remaining services, still at ECH, onto our DGH hospital campus.
In due course it became apparent that cancer services would be first in line – mainly because it was a net earner for the hospital, whereas A&E typically operated at a loss because the tariff attached to A&E attenders was totally inadequate.
After becoming a Governor I pressed for management to give us details about where this new radiotherapy department would be built, mindful of the fact that if it was built in the wrong location it would compromise any eventual emergency services reprovision.
In the autumn 0f 2011 the Governors were given a presentation by the Director of Operations.

She was a qualified pharmacist, who had played a crucial part in the downfall of Slough's Wexham Park Hospital.

Her presentation gave no real details about the content of this new department, apart from the chosen site being the unoccupied space between the original DGH building and the Gainsborough Wing. In my mind this location would have been

166

ideal for any new ED, and there was at least one other site on the hospital campus where the Radiotherapy Department could be built, and where one of the original bidders for our PFI had placed it.

After that meeting I resurrected some comprehensive architectural drawings which I had presented to our MAC soon after our PFI had been abandoned. These plans showed how not only the new radiotherapy department, but also the ED, some extra ward capacity as well as the Pathology Services, which everyone had forgotten about, could be included in the same building.

Immediately before our next Governors' Council meeting I booked a room in our Postgraduate Centre to show my proposals to a selected group of Governors, so that when we were eventually shown the definitive plans we would have some informed opinions about other alternatives.

A few days later our SIC discovered that I had convened this meeting, and a previous meeting without her 'permission'. Greatly annoyed she officially cancelled the meeting, but decided that in future there would be a short private session of Governors prior to each monthly Governors' Council meeting.

Then I arranged a meeting with SIC, which incidentally she enthusiastically agreed to attend, in order to show her my alternative strategy, but at the last minute she claimed that she had a stomach bug.

That meeting was cancelled and never reconvened!

At the next public meeting of the Governors' Council the actual plans for the new radiotherapy department had been put on as the last item on the agenda, but this item had not been added to the agenda of the preceding Governors' private meeting, in spite of my efforts, and that of another Governor, to include it.

The agendas were duly circulated a few days before those meetings. Now the only way to discuss those radiotherapy plans would be under Any Other Business (AOB).

The private meeting took place, but it was almost entirely occupied by the Lead Governor raising some issues about how the Governors' Code of Practice might be modified. That did not leave enough time in AOB for the radiotherapy paper to be discussed!

So we all went into the following public meeting without a plan on how we could change or even sabotage the Board's plan for the new radiotherapy department.

These public meetings took place in a large room with the Governors, NEDs and some Board members arranged around a ring doughnut shaped table, with our SIC at the head.

Members of the general public sat around the walls of the room. Board members, who had items on the agenda gave their presentation followed by questions from those present, but questions were skilfully controlled by our SIC.

The Director of Finance usually gave an appraisal of the Trust's financial position, and tried to explain how they would deliver efficiency savings.

Year on year efficiency savings were an essential remit for every FHT, and had been imposed in order to meet spending targets, but they were supposed to represent a long-term reduction in outgoings, whereas in reality the Board used 'temporary' cut backs in staffing, especially under-resourcing the nursing establishment.

This public meeting progressed at a snail's pace.

People started to fidget and look at the clock.

Finally the last item on the agenda came up and I was quick to start the questions, but after only a few weak replies from the Director of Operations, our SIC cut me short and said that other people should have their say.

Some rather irrelevant questions were asked, and that signalled the end of the proceedings.

There was no vote or other mechanism put in place to make amendments to the plans on the table.

Our SIC then closed the session saying words to effect 'well I take it that that is agreed'!

I was livid, as were a few of my Governor colleagues who had seen and understood my alternative plans. One of these was an engineer who had compiled a list of problems with the Trust's plans, but who had been denied the opportunity to speak. Furthermore there was a judicial review in the pipeline questioning the rationale for increasing the number of Linear Accelerators in Colchester's Radiotherapy plans, when it would have been more patient friendly to have built a small radiotherapy centre in Chelmsford (Mid Essex).

On the following day I emailed our Medical Director, pointing out the deficiencies and errors in the calculations in the documents which had been presented, and which we had apparently agreed to, asking him to intervene or at least give the Governors an opportunity to have a meaningful conversation. Then I copied this email to two erstwhile medical colleagues at the hospital.

Within twenty four hours I received a reprimand from our SIC saying that I had overstepped the terms and conditions laid out in the Governors' code of practice, because I had communicated with hospital employees without first getting permission to do so via the Membership office, and had in her eyes made a libellous accusation about the Director of Operations and her sidekick!

After that I received a flurry of emails from other Governors giving me their support, but a disciplinary meeting was nonetheless set up for the following month with a view to dismissing me as a Governor.

I was told to write an apology to the Director of Operations and her sidekick, and also told that at the extraordinary meeting of the Governors' Council which would follow, my misdemeanour would be discussed (in my absence) and without my being able to question any of the Governors, and in particular any Governor whom I suspected had leaked my emails to our SIC.

That meeting was duly held in December, where I was given a dressing down, and then had to recite an apology to the meeting which had been **written for me** by the Director of Human Resources.

Well – talk about the reincarnation of the Star Chamber!

169

The only reason why I wasn't sacked for that offence, was because a substantial body of Governors had defended my actions!

After that I contacted the Chairman of Monitor, who fobbed me off with, 'it was none of their business, and that I should bring the affair to the attention of our NED's Senior Independent Director (SID)'.

Our SID just told me that complaints had to come through the Lead Governor after discussion at a Governors' Council meeting!

Fat chance, with the Lead Governor in our SIC's pocket!

Then I contacted Harriet Messenger, who had been the leading light at that FTGA meeting in July 2011, but she had no power to discipline our SIC.

From now on, and with my card marked, I clearly had to watch my P's and Q's

However, my obsessional commitment, to get the Emergency Service moved up the agenda, soon got me in hot water again.

What I needed was the support of our A&E Consultant, who was an interim appointment as a result of the Colchester Garrison seconding him to the hospital.

The incumbent was a Surgeon with the rank of Major, but with little concept of how the NHS operated. He thrived on a diet of major surgical incidents, but was nonplussed by the usual flood of medical, mainly geriatric, referrals.

In my simplistic mind I thought that a military allegory might appeal to him and spark some enthusiasm.

Unfortunately, I should have tried to get to know him better before presenting him with a Daniel DeFoeesque allegory.

My plan backfired. My allegory had merely confused him and he just passed it on to our SIC, who jumped at the opportunity to finally get her own way, and get rid of me, more especially now since I had contacted Monitor about her behaviour.

The subsequent disciplinary meeting in March 2012 followed the previous format, once again without me being able to say anything in my defence,

Some time later, this Military A&E Consultant was 'discharged', after he had thrown a tantrum and trashed his office. Had I realised that he was a bit of an oddball, I might not have written that allegory!

My departure left me ruing my decision to resign as a Governor to Ipswich Hospital, but I was still determined to try and put some of my extensive medical experience to good use.

That opportunity would arise in 2014 when new Governor elections were to be held.

In the meantime I put my name forward for election as a public member of the Health Forum Committee (HFC) of our recently created CCG – the new iteration of our PCT.

With the advent of new Governor elections, I requested the necessary application forms from the hospital's Membership Office, but after having waited for almost two weeks for the required documentation to arrive and the deadline for applications drawing close, I contacted a friendly member of staff, who had some clout in the real hospital. She swiftly forwarded the forms to me and I submitted them to the external electoral body which was carrying out the election process. However, with less than eight hours to the deadline, I received an email from the electoral body saying that my application was invalid because my name was not on the Membership List. I immediately contacted my friendly member of staff again. She replied that she would look into this curious business, and just after lunch the same day I received her reply, in which she confirmed that somebody must have removed my name from the list of Members, and that she had reinstated me with a new membership number.

I contacted the electoral body with these details and just before 17.00 I received a reply from them saying that my application was now valid!

I was duly re-elected only to discover that in the interim my friendly member of staff had been dismissed from the Trust, on the grounds that there had been some inaccuracies in her

Curriculum Vitae when she had originally been appointed, and that made her appointment invalid!!

Guess who put the knife in?

I felt sorry that I had been responsible for this, but could find no way in which I could contact her and offer my apologies, and the Human Resources department would not give me her forwarding address.

No surprise there!

The handful of activist Governors, who had been members of the Council for the last six years, had not applied for re-election. Therefore in future disputes with our SIC I was likely to be standing alone.

The first business of our new Council was to elect a Lead Governor. Several names were put forward, including my own, but the person elected did not come from our hospital's catchment area, but from 'the rest of Essex'. He was a paramedic, so at least he would understand the needs of our emergency service, but the whole point of having Governors had been the need to have local public representation, and he was not local!

My new term of office with the Governors' Council coincided with the replacement of our previous CEO.

The new CEO had been parachuted in to help us out of Special Measures. She was an attractive young lady who came with her *Curriculum Vitae* full of accolades, and in particular her achievements as a senior nurse.

Our SIC had had little say in this appointment, unlike the appointment of GCE our previous CEO, where her role seemed to have been pivotal.

GCE had been a senior executive of Big Pharma, and then in his retirement had looked for something worthwhile to occupy his time. It is unclear why he had put his name forward for our vacant CEO post because, just like our

SIC, he did not live in our district, and his only previous experience in the NHS had been a couple of years as a junior doctor.

It soon became apparent that he was out of his depth, as CHUFT tried to grapple with meeting the national clinical waiting time targets. Then when the director of our MAU invited me to attend a meeting where the future of our emergency services were to be discussed, I thought that the Board had finally become clinically focussed but, on arriving, GCE asked me to leave because as far as he was concerned, it was a <u>private</u> meeting!

Big Pharma might operate in that way, but the NHS had been founded on collaboration and not aggressive competition!

It did not take GCE long to lead the Board into an impossible meltdown, which resulted in CHUFT being placed into Special Measures.

Now we had another new CEO at the head of our organisation who knew something about healthcare. Clearly her remit had been to move the hospital forward so that we could be taken out of Special Measures.

She came across as someone who cared about patients, but within the first month of her appointment it was apparent to me from our SIC's body language, at our public meetings that for her, the new CEO was *persona non grata*.

This clash of personalities lasted for about three months when this brilliant nurse CEO resigned!

Why could nobody see that our SIC was destroying the hospital's credibility?

At one of the Governors' Council public meetings, a member of the public asked our SIC why she had not resigned when the cancer waiting times scandal had erupted. Her answer was evasive and gave the impression that she did not understand the question. It was the Governors who had the power to call for her removal not the public, and the lemming-like Governors were totally under her thumb!

Another new CEO was parachuted in – LMCE. She had been the CEO of Whipps Cross Hospital, and had overseen the hospital's downgrading as part of the financial package to help the Barts/London Hospital FHT out of a financial black hole.

LMCE was a timid person, and putty in the hands of our SIC.

Soon after this there was another appointment to the Board.

The incumbent's title was 'Secretary' but not in the usual sense of that description.

Her role was to assist in the process of getting the hospital out of Special Measures, and she set about her task by arranging a series of one to one interviews with all the members of the Board, the NEDs and the Governors.

This was quite a reasonable start for someone trying to get to the bottom of the hospital's dysfunctional management.

I found my interview with her to be very searching and thorough, and I looked forward to the end of the hospital's horrible past.

Unsurprisingly there was discord on the Board.

It was felt that her terms of reference had been misinterpreted by her.

The Director of Operations then sent a confidential email to *'everyone concerned'* saying this new member of the Trust had been fired.

This breath of fresh air had been snuffed out – just like that!

On the following day I received a telephone call from one of the journalists on the Colchester Gazette, in which he asked me if the sacking of this person was true. Naturally I gave him an affirmative answer, although I was curious why he had asked me when he clearly already had the answer. In the subsequent conversation I probably added a little more about the real problem on the Board – namely our SIC.

The journalist then published his 'scoop' in the Colchester Gazette, but included my name – maybe to give it some authenticity. However, that was like a red rag to a bull, and our SIC immediately called another disciplinary meeting, because in her words I had contacted a journalist without first clearing it with the hospital's public relations officer.

The fact that it had been the journalist who had contacted me and not the other way around, did not concern our SIC.

Once again she had me by the short and curlies, but on this occasion it just constituted a first warning. I also realised that I

174

could no longer rely upon the support of those activist Governors, who were now no longer on the Governors' Council.

Any further infringement of the code of practice would be fatal. Our SIC didn't have to wait long for that.

Outsourcing Pathology Services
When it comes to deciding NHS policy, the bean counters are the top dogs and appear to be able to overrule all clinical objections.

A prime example of this was the way in which laboratory services were destroyed by the centralisation hub and spoke principle enshrined in the Carter Report.

Carter was a businessman who chaired a number of committees charged with reducing the cost of critical government services.

The 2003 report on prison services was conducted on the basis of adopting a *'credible and effective system, which is focused on reducing crime and maintaining public confidence, whilst remaining affordable'*, but needless to say it was the effect on 'affordability' which dominated the outcome.

In 2008 Carter's Report on pathology services was published, but in spite of it meeting pretty universal opposition from the Pathologists, it was being successively rolled out across the country. Its main flaw was that as the hub increased in size, so the spokes would become unable to provide an effective emergency service.

The NHS had succeeded in scoring one of its biggest own goals!

This effect had been predicted from the very start, but objections were systematically overruled. This meant that in 2019 when the Coronavirus pandemic hit the UK, the system was unfit for purpose and unable to support any attempt by those left in Public Health to monitor, identify or trace contacts.

For Colchester it meant that all our biological samples would in future be processed at Ipswich Hospital.

175

The laboratory service providers at Basildon Hospital had kicked up a fuss when they heard that their hub would be in Cambridge, and then made their own arrangements to set up a hub closer to home.

Back in Colchester I met with a group of our own hospital laboratory staff over lunch, and when I realised that they were totally against this move, I said that I would try to get it reversed or at least made into a more acceptable package.

By this time I was an HFC member of our CCG. In that role I highlighted the problems that outsourcing laboratory services would create, and also voiced them when I attended another of the CCGs subcommittees which was in discussions with a proposed service provider.

One of its systematic flaws was how blood cultures and samples of Cerebrospinal Fluid (CSF) would be handled expeditiously.

At a subsequent meeting of the HFC, I was given the task of probing CHUFT for their Board's opinion on this matter.

Emboldened by my research and the concern of my HFC colleagues, I asked for the issue to be put on the agenda of the next Governors' briefings by LMCE and SIC.

This had long been a regular weekly morning meeting with the CEO and our SIC. These meetings were usually quite informative, although they rarely revealed anything which we did not already know, and typically only a handful of Governors bothered to attend.

However, two months passed without this issue being discussed, and as a result I emailed the Medical Director, who was one of the hospital's two Microbiologists, in order to find out what CHUFT was proposing to do.

I received a guarded reply from the Medical Director and then a barbed email from our SIC.

Once again I had contravened the Code of Practice by contacting a member of staff without first getting prior permission from the Membership Office!

Another extraordinary meeting of the Governors' Council was convened, and I was duly sacked without being able to explain my position to the assembled Governors.

176

Now I really had had enough.

The FHT Governor deception was totally unfit for purpose, and nothing short of a new act of Parliament was likely to change it.

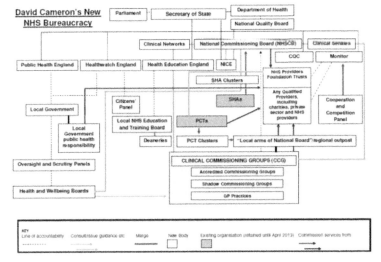

Blueprint for Lansley's 2012 HSC Act

22

The CCG Health Forum Committee

Not long after I had been sacked for the first time as a Governor at CHUFT, the recently formed NE Essex CCG, invited their catchment population, who were registered with a North East Essex General Practice, to apply for posts on their HFC.

Our CCG had just replaced the PCT as the finite purchaser of healthcare services for the local community. The management structure of these CCGs was much smaller than that of the PCTs and had an executive committee with a majority of local GPs. In the meantime, the redundant members of the erstwhile local PCT set up their own business, Anglia Community Enterprise (ACE), offering services to the local community, and in due course the CCG purchased those services from ACE.

ACE was in effect a private consortium which still used the NHS logo on their communications (illegally), so it looked as though everything had not changed, but ACE's profits were not necessarily reinvested in the NHS!

By and large CCGs had the impossible task of commissioning care with a reduced budget and the extra expense of putting virtually every item of care out to tender. Common sense would have encouraged them to renew contracts with historically reliable providers, but that carried the risk of being challenged by interested parties, which had almost bottomless pockets to fight a rejected tender through the courts.

This was in fact a cross between commercial blackmail and bullying!

I put my name forward, and was duly elected onto the HFC.

The HFC consisted of about a dozen members of the local community, most of whom had had personal experience of NHS treatment.

From amongst its members, the HFC elected their own Chairman in a secret ballot.

I had been one of three contenders, but came bottom in the election.

179

The HFC Chairman, or the deputy, was charged with representing our committee's opinions at the CCG's public Board meetings. This was quite onerous, since these meetings often lasted more than four hours.

We held our own public meetings with some of the items on each agenda having been requested by members of the public. Additionally, each HFC member was allotted a number of General Practice Surgeries, which they were expected to engage with, and attend the practice's support group meetings.

The practice support group members were like hospital Governors, except that those wishing to be involved had to be approved by the doctors running the practice.

We also sat in on various CCG subcommittees, and then reported back at the next private session of the HFC.

This inclusivity was in stark contrast to the dumbed down way in which CHUFT treated their Governors!

The public really was having a say about which services the CCG would fund, and the quality of those services funded, but there was an underlying financial handicap imposed by the 2012 HSC Act.

In June 2014, at a meeting of our CCG, the nature of the neck-lock constraining our CCG was revealed.

Our catchment population was just over 300,000 with more than the national average of people over the age of 60.

Our budget, which came from NHS England (NHSE), was £412m, but we had to make 'efficiency/productivity' savings of £18m year on year, which meant that in 2015 the budget would likely be £394m and £376m in 2016!

With this reducing budget we were expected amongst other considerations to commission services to deliver 'Care Closer to Home', and enhance our 'Urgent Care' and 'End of Life' performance.

As young doctors, even with both hands tied behind our backs, we would have bent over backwards to achieve the 'impossible', but **this** was ridiculous!

Patient Choice

Public consultation and patient choice are two aspects of democracy which can result in unexpected and not necessarily beneficial outcomes to the community or the individual patient. The quantity, quality and truthfulness of the information given before that choice is made can be critical, and may be used by the dishonest to distort the decision-making process in their favour. Another word for this practice is propaganda.

Although democracy, at least in theory, gives the democratized community choice, choice expects those with choice to be responsible in the way in which they exercise this privilege, but also accept being responsible for the outcome.

By and large our choices depend upon what we can afford, but when given a free health service, people seem to think that they could demand virtually anything.

In 1945 the people chose a socialist agenda.

In 1951 the people chose a return to a capitalist economy.

Our forebears made those choices, but they did not live long enough to reap the harvest.

Short-sightedness is as much the legacy of the voting public as it is of the scheming politicians whom we choose to make the decisions that rule our lives.

In the 2005 False-Labour Party General Election manifesto, Tony Blair, the pseudo-socialist undeclared capitalist Prime Minister, promised to give NHS patients more choice, and in 2007 the details emerged. However, as was usually the case, the politicians had failed to address the small print issue of how this enhancement would be funded.

Saying that patients would in future be able to choose where to have their treatment, if the local facility was unable to deliver within an agreed time frame, and promising to deliver care closer to the patient's home, was little more than a ploy to win votes at the election.

Little headway was made on this promise over the next five years, but there had been some catastrophic financial world events to cope with.

When the voters went to the polls again in 2010, no party had an overall majority, but a power sharing deal with the Liberal Democrats allowed the Conservative Party to take back the reins from the Labour Party.

The Liberal Democrats in this coalition had clearly abandoned their liberal roots, and their capitalist leader, relishing the opportunity to go to bed with David Cameron, allowed the most outrageous 2012 Healthcare Bill to become law.

Patient choice, which had temporarily been lost in this bloody bathwater, re-emerged, but without addressing the question of funding, other than the belief that it would come out of efficiency savings, and promote the opportunity of different deliverers of healthcare to compete with each other for the associated tariffs, and thereby reshape the geography of healthcare. Telling patients that they could receive their healthcare – general practice and hospital attendances – wherever they wished to go, was rolled out in the hope that patients 'voting with their feet' would give the overlords the opportunity to close certain local services.

All it did was to create confusion.

If you were IT literate, then in theory you could make an appointment on a date and time of your choosing with any hospital consultant anywhere in the country, provided that you had a letter of referral from your chosen GP.

Also, provided that your chosen surgery had given you a specific password, you could book an appointment with any care professional at your local surgery or health centre.

Were these 'new' developments worth the effort, and was this not yet another diversionary tactic to take our eyes off the real political agenda?

Before the NHS came into force, patient choice was simply a matter of general knowledge of the medical landscape, and the size of your wallet, although it still might have been your chosen GP who made the initial 'specialist' recommendation.

After 1948, patient choice became clouded by the way in which patients were cross-referred between specialties without the patient playing much part in the process.

Sometimes this turned out well, but this was not the rule.

I will illustrate this dilemma with two different aspects of patient choice.

1. In the autumn of 1965, Joseph Isaacs was admitted as an emergency to Mile End Hospital suffering from jaundice.

From the patient's history, physical examination and laboratory tests, it was apparent that he had obstructive jaundice and the likely cause was cancer of the head of the pancreas.

Dr Dolphin (my boss) asked one of our Surgeons to see Mr Isaacs.

We gathered around the patient's bed, and waited as our diagnosis was confirmed.

The Surgeon looked Mr Isaacs squarely in the face and explained that the next step would be an operation to relieve the obstruction.

Mr Isaacs said nothing.

I spoke to his wife and explained the nature of the underlying disease and the need for surgery.

She agreed with our decision, but at no stage did she or any of us tell the patient that he probably had cancer.

Mr Isaacs had his own small shoe repair shop just off the Mile End Road, and by all accounts was not a wealthy man, but one wonders what he might have done before 1948. More likely than not, he would have chosen one of the Surgeons at the London Jewish Hospital, which was just around the corner in Stepney Green.

On the following day I asked Mr Isaacs to sign the operation consent form.

He spent a long time reading and re-reading the text.

His choice was either to sign, or not to sign.

He chose not to sign, and at the same time asked for a second opinion!

What a dilemma!

The operation was cancelled, and Dr Dolphin asked Professor Sheila Sherlock, from the Royal Free Hospital, to give that 'second opinion'.

A couple of days later, Professor Sherlock with her retinue, which included her chief assistant, rolled up.

Along with the ward sister there must have been about six doctors assembled around Mr Isaac's bed.

It took Professor Sherlock, a rather dogmatic woman who did not suffer fools gladly, no time at all to concur with our diagnosis, and tell the patient that he needed an operation.

Mr Isaacs said nothing, but after the entourage had gone, he told me that he wanted another opinion!

183

I spent some time with his wife explaining that the jaundice and intractable itch would be relieved by the operation, although it would probably not cure the underlying disease.

She must have convinced her husband of the need for surgery as soon as possible, and then she signed the consent form on his behalf.

Sure enough, within a few days of the operation the jaundice was beginning to fade and the itch had all but gone. His appetite returned, and he began to eat the kosher meals provided by the hospital kitchen.

(All patients could choose from a menu which included – diabetic, weight reduction, vegetarian, and kosher. So he was able to make some choices!)

After the sutures had been removed, he returned home, but was readmitted semi-comatose a couple of months later.

My guess is that he would have chosen not to be readmitted to hospital, but events overtook him and he died not in a place of his own choice.

Our hospital, like all hospitals, was an island, and we had no control over what emergency patients washed up on our shore.

2. Early in the 1990s, a young French teacher, from the local grammar school, was referred to my outpatient clinic with thyrotoxicosis.

She had had several months of treatment with Carbimazole (the drug of choice at that time), and the condition was well under control.

Her GP had suggested that the time had come to 'cure' her disease, and hence the referral.

I explained all the pros and cons of the way forward, which included surgery, radioactive iodine, or long-term Carbimazole therapy.

My recommendation was for radioactive iodine.

I gave her a copy of the guidelines which I had already explained to her, and asked her to return on the following week with her decision.

She chose surgery, but qualified that by asking if I could recommend a good surgeon.

For some reason she was not happy with having the operation in Colchester.

Maybe she had heard about the two fatalities which had occurred over the past couple of decades.

There are a number of side-effects of surgery for thyrotoxicosis other than death from thyroid storm. The most disabling is hypoparathyroidism resulting from the inadvertent removal of the parathyroid glands. These are usually four in number, very small and embedded in the thyroid itself.

I recommended a Surgeon at St Thomas' Hospital in London. He had been my choice of Surgeon for the removal of an overactive parathyroid adenoma.

Surely, I had said to myself, that he would first identify the parathyroid glands and then make a strenuous attempt to avoid their removal.

Unfortunately, that turned out not to be the case!

So this young lady's choice turned out to be a long-term millstone around her neck, with her having to juggle the treatment for both hypothyroidism and hypoparathyroidism.

The latter is always the more difficult to control.

Clearly giving the choice to the patient has serious flaws.

Had she been a teenager, I would have chosen the treatment and, with the support of her parent or guardian, probably prescribed radioactive iodine.

The downside, of the doctor making the choice, is that if everything does not go according to plan, then the doctor could be sued!

The NHS choice agenda did nothing to make patient choice any easier or more appropriate.

The patient could now choose where to go for hospital treatment and even choose the date and time of that appointment, but could not choose the doctor.

That was only possible in the Private Sector.

Going back to our CCG.

I was asked to form a subcommittee to address the subject of 'Patient Choice', and chair its meetings. After many deliberations we eventually reached a consensus, and an informative leaflet was printed to explain the 'rights' of the public, and point out the potential disadvantages of seeking medical care outside our locality.

I also sat on the CCG's R&D Committee, which probed with a great sense of commitment into what the CCG expected of those bidding to provide services, and then be legally bound to follow. From here a subcommittee was set up to examine the tenders from those providers wishing to deliver diabetes care in the community, and I was invited to give advice.

Over many decades in NE Essex there had been a long-running difference of opinion about whether or not diabetics in our locality had a higher than average rate of limb amputation. This formed one of the reasons why our PCT decided to appoint a Diabetologist whose contract included improving diabetes services in our community.

In 2013 our CCG used the English national data, from 158 PCTs relating to amputations carried out from 2007-2010, in order to act as a guide to appointing the provider of diabetes services in NE Essex.

CHUFT lacked a bespoke Diabetes Centre, and we were jealous of the provision of this service at Ipswich Hospital. Getting the contract for the community diabetes service in NE Essex might have given us the opportunity to build our own facility. In fact we had toyed with the idea of setting it up in the new PCT building just down the road, but at the time there had been insufficient space available. However with the CCG now only occupying about half of the upper floor of their premises, this opportunity was rekindled.

With the CCG concentrating on foot care, rather than our excellent results from our combined O&G and Diabetes pregnancy service, we might have been at a disadvantage. Furthermore the CHUFT submission contained a glaringly obvious error relating to our costs of providing that service.

There were two entries relating to the joint diabetes and obstetrics clinic, and these had different HRG codes. One code was an O&G code, and the other one was a General Medical code. With the tariff system of hospital remuneration, each patient episode which carried either code entitled the hospital to claim the appropriate level of remuneration from the PCT (now the CCG).

In practical terms the remuneration was the means whereby individual departments could obtain funding for their services. However the invoice from the O&G Directorate was identical to the invoice submitted by the Medical Directorate, when clearly only one patient episode had taken place.

One wonders how many other devious manoeuvres were being accidentally or fraudulently used by the finance departments of other hospitals.

I don't know whether or not this played a part in the awarding of the contract, because these were confidential matters, and not shared with anyone outside the Board of Directors.

The hospital did not get the contract, which was a pity, but the hospital lacked the tendering skills of the Private Sector!

It is also a pity that the commissioners and providers of healthcare had to engage in this adversarial way, although it was supposed to ensure that services were tailored to the needs of the local population, but within the available budget allocated to the CCG by central government.

Confidentiality

One of the other differences, between the CCG and the local hospital, was the way in which confidential or sensitive material was handled.

In the CCG office, to which HFC members had free access, the only sensitive information was in the details of the bids of those competing for vacant contracts, and this was not in the public domain, whereas within the hospital environment sensitive information was everywhere.

There were lists of employees, and readily accessible lists of patients waiting to attend the outpatient department, or undergo investigative or surgical procedures.

The most sensitive documents were the patients' case notes, which used to be everywhere in plain sight for anyone to pick up and peruse. This could be a great hunting ground for busybodies and social deviants to access information inappropriately.

Trusting in people's honesty was never going to be a good ploy! It was therefore perfectly reasonable only to allow Governors access to the hospital when accompanied by an accredited senior hospital employee or NED.

There is another side to confidentiality which has very blurred edges.

For example, when a whistle blower exposes confidential material, he risks his job and future employability, but an investigative journalist, who obtains employment with a view to filming the abuse of patients by healthcare staff, risks nothing.

Was the nurse, who reported her Consultant for facilitating the death of a patient, breaching confidentiality?

When a doctor allows the police to access a patient's private space, before the police have obtained the necessary Court Order, is that a breach of confidentiality?

I found myself in this difficult position several years ago, when two sisters, rescued from a house fire at night, were admitted as emergencies with carbon monoxide poisoning.

The elder woman, who had chronic lung disease, probably from lifelong cigarette smoking, had blood carbon monoxide levels three times lower than her fit looking sister, who was found on admission to have severe bronchial mucosal necrosis from the inhalation of smoke,

This was especially curious since they shared the same bedroom.

One of the investigating police officers approached me saying that he suspected arson, and that the elder sister had probably played some part. Furthermore the family – a grandparent, two parents and the two sisters - had recently been made homeless in the Midlands, where the property they had occupied had been trashed. On arriving in Clacton, Social Services had found them a two bedroom flat, but the family demanded something bigger. According to the police the only breadwinner in this dysfunctional family was the younger sister, who had found employment as a shop assistant.

Apparently, with a member of the family earning money, that reduced the pecking order of the family for better accommodation.

When I heard this tale I was incensed, because by then the younger sister had died. I allowed the police to fit a listening device in the single room occupied by the elder sister, when she was away having a chest x-ray. The police then listened in to conversations between the patient and her relatives, from a command vehicle parked two floors below in a courtyard.

Later I was told that no useful oral information had been obtained, but that might have been a cover to let me off the hook.

In retrospect, the police could quite easily have found a way of inserting that bug without involving me or my ward sister, but time had been of the essence.

Patient confidentiality is extremely complex and it was not resolved by the appointment of Caldicott Guardians, who were put in impossible situations if there was a Police Investigation. This was tested in Colchester, when a whistleblower created a legal challenge to CHUFT, because proof of wrongdoing would require access to patients' case notes.

In 2015, after three years on the CCG's HFC, I decided not to put my name up for re-election. I felt that I was leaving our future care in good hands, although I did detect some frustration with the system. Doctors in general usually find a way of solving problems even in adverse situations, but doctors don't like to be **told** what to do, especially by their colleagues, after all, GPs on CCGs only represented about 5% of the local GP force.

Why should we be **told** where to buy paper clips, and who should provide community nursing services?

Elsewhere in the UK satisfaction with local CCGs was less rosy. In places GPs formed less than 50% of the Board and clearly no longer had control of which services were purchased.

Meaningful Redress

In 1974, the True-Labour government of Harold Wilson set up Community Health Councils (CHCs), and this was enhanced by the Community Health Councils Access to Information Act (1988). Half of the members were appointed by local authorities, a third by local voluntary organisations and a sixth by the RHA, which provided the finance to pay staff and costs. They were entitled to be consulted on any substantial development of the health service, and on any proposals to make a substantial variation in the service.

CHCs were very effective in challenging inappropriate policies such as the closure of Edgware Hospital in Greater London and Kidderminster Hospital in the Midlands.

In 2008 the False-Labour government of Tony Blair abolished CHCs and replaced them with a succession of toothless impotent alternatives such as Healthwatch.

Community Councils were first established in Scotland following the Local Government (Scotland) Act 1973. Thereafter, the Local Government (Scotland) Act, 1994, which produced the current system of unitary local authorities, made provision for the continuation of community councils. Under this legislation, every local community in Scotland is entitled to petition their local authority to establish a community council in their area. Wales followed a similar strategy.

Public consultation on new healthcare initiatives in England reached a peak of absurdity when Ara Darzi, a Professor of minimal invasive surgical techniques at London's Imperial College, was asked in 2007 to sound out public opinion on the modernisation of the NHS, first in London and then in the rest of England.

By some curious twist of fate I found myself invited to attend one of these meetings at the Department of Health, along with a few doctors and nurses and a whole host of other seemingly random participants drawn from the English shires.

Mr Darzi arrived late, gave a presentation and left early. Someone from the DoH, whose name I cannot remember, stood in to answer questions, but gave little reassurance that our concerns would be addressed.

The best part of a day wasted on this farce!

It 'validated' the decision to set up Polyclinics financed not by new money but by withdrawing funding from other parts of the NHS.

When David Cameron, Nick Clegg, Andrew Lansley and their cronies took over the NHS rudder, they had already had an important bit of meaningless spadework done for them by False-Labour!

23

Public Health

Both before and immediately after 1948, Public Health was funded by local taxes raised from the householders and businesses which in turn elected the Borough and County Councillors, who were charged with delivering appropriate Public Health services to the local community.

At the end of each financial year, the Council had to send a report to the Ministry detailing a breakdown of local health concerns, and a tally of the notifiable diseases recorded.

In March 1949 the Health Ministry produced a very upbeat account of the state of health of the nation, and lauded the success of the NHS in the significant reduction of notifiable diseases such as influenza and tuberculosis. However, the winter of 1948 had been particularly mild, and along with other factors, the idea that the introduction of the NHS in July 1948 had been responsible, was rather premature.

Nonetheless this was an auspicious start.

Right from the start there had been disagreement in the Labour cabinet about whether Public Health should remain as a locally driven engine for health improvement, or as a vassal for government driven directives. Nye Bevan had feared that left to their own devices, local health boards in the Tory heartlands would just pocket the financial support from the government, and reduce the level of local taxation.

Unsurprisingly Nye adopted a top down Public Health Agenda, whilst retaining local Medical Officers for Health, their operational staff and laboratory infrastructure.

In this situation the identification and contact tracing of people infected with any of the notifiable diseases would remain robust, and a bulwark against runaway epidemics.

The government plans, to reduce early childhood mortality, were organised from local health centres where free cod liver oil and concentrated orange juice were handed out, and schedules of immunization initiated.

All school children were given $^1/_3$ pint free milk daily until 1968 when Harold Wilson confined it to primary schools, and in 1971 Margaret Thatcher cut it out altogether, but by then early childhood mortality had been almost 'eliminated'.

Cleaning up the environment was another task for the local Public Health committees, and great strides were made over the following decades to reduce air pollution and the pollution of the waterways, but new pollutants were continually being introduced into the environment, and keeping track of these was a headache for all concerned.

The discovery of asbestos with its unique non-flammable insulating properties lead to its widespread use in the construction industry, but its elimination from the built environment in Britain only became an ongoing task for the MOH during the NHS era.

The elimination of environmental pollution by lead, from the lead tetra ethyl added to petroleum, was a national success story, and unleaded petrol became the norm.

Fluorinated hydrocarbons like trichlorofluoromethane had been introduced as aerosol propellants and refrigerants to replace flammable alternatives, but these were eventually implicated in depleting the ozone layer in the atmosphere, and a factor in global warming. Subsequent legislation sorted that out.

With the budget for Public Health just part of the local community's remit, there was always the risk that other areas of council spending could siphon off resources from Public Health and make it less able to cope with unexpected health problems.

Many councils were aware of this handicap, and ring fenced their Public Health budgets. Others were less cautious.

Another of the many Public Health initiatives introduced in the 1940s had been the promotion of the use of Mass Miniature Radiography (MMR) for the detection of pulmonary tuberculosis in asymptomatic people, and those who had been in close contact with tuberculous patients. The subsequent isolation in sanatoria of those affected, was intended to reduce the spread of Tuberculosis (TB) in the community, but apart from bed rest, a nutritious diet, fresh air and actinotherapy (exposure to UV light), there weren't any specific antibacterial treatments.

With the discovery of Streptomycin in 1944, Para-aminosalicylic acid in 1946, and Isoniazid in 1952, there was a real chance that TB could be cured, and screening using MMR became more than just a tool to record the prevalence of TB. However, false positive findings could expose patients to the hazards of chemotherapy, and the drug treatment of TB was not without significant risks.

In 1963, a factory in Slough had their employees screened for TB using a visiting MMR facility. Only one member of staff, Mr Lightfoot, had what was thought to be a positive MMR, and he was referred to the local chest physician.

It was ironic that this man's future medical problem should be related in his surname!

In due course Mr Lightfoot was admitted to our chest ward in Taplow. However, in spite of sputum, throat swabs and gastric washings yielding no evidence of TB, triple chemotherapy was started.

After one month the patient developed a mild fever.

An adverse drug reaction was suspected, and all treatment was stopped.

Within a couple of days the fever had abated, and on the assumption that para-aminosalicylic acid had been the culprit, treatment with streptomycin alone was restarted.

Within an hour of the streptomycin injection, Mr Lightfoot 'collapsed'.

He was pale, his blood pressure was barely recordable, and he complained of pain in the buttock which had received the injection.

The foot of the bed was raised and he was given some Pethidine for the pain.

Soon his blood pressure had risen satisfactorily, and the pain in the buttock had improved.

Nonetheless the foot of the bed remained raised by about half a metre.

Over the course of the rest of the day and especially during the night, the patient continued to complain of pain, and repeated injections of Pethidine were given without anyone examining his legs.

In fact the pain was by then in both feet and not in his buttock!

In the morning when the bedclothes were pulled back, several toes from both feet were found to be cyanosed or black.

The upshot was that prolonged exposure of his feet to a low blood pressure, exacerbated by the elevation of his legs and the hypotensive effects of Pethidine had resulted in ischaemic necrosis of several toes and part of his forefoot, which subsequently required amputation.

Underlying arterial disease may have been an important factor, but without this adverse drug reaction and inappropriate management thereof, his feet might have remained intact for many years.

This is just one case in which Public Health screening unfortunately went wrong, but there are many other diseases, particularly in the screening for breast cancer, where a Danish study claimed that, except where a lump had previously been identified, screening could do more harm than good.

Nonetheless, the successes of Public Health initiatives in the discovery of overt treatable diseases should not be belittled. However, the investigation and treatment of those in whom the actual cause of a disease is far from clear, is an area of disease prevention where extreme caution in needed.

For those of us who had experienced better joined up working practices and cared about the future sustainability of the NHS, we had let the substance of healthcare slip through our fingers and were left impotent to reverse the train as it ploughed on regardless.

If we had really cared, we could have stood on the tracks barring the juggernaut's progress, but we stepped aside and took retirement and a generous pension instead.

The Coronavirus Pandemic
It took the appearance of Covid-19 on our doorstep, for the slashers of Public Health to realise their folly.

The year on year reduction in the NHS budget, the loss of hospital beds, the selling of NHS real-estate to the Private

196

Sector and the employment of the Private Sector to deliver healthcare, all contributed to the lack of facilities available to deal with a major disaster when the Coronavirus arrived in the UK.

An event like this, which is only likely to strike once in a century, should not mean that we should be unprepared for it. Had so much of the family silver not been sold, we would probably have been able to cope and effectively contain the epidemic.

New Zealand's socialist government acted swiftly, and by temporarily shutting down their economy and concentrating on disease containment, their efforts should have served as a lesson for all capitalist economies to follow.

Initially New Zealand's Prime Minister was severely criticised and temporarily became extremely unpopular, but the success of her action has now earned her massive popularity and unending gratitude from her people.

British economists were quick to point out that had we retained the entire infrastructure inherited in 1948, the cost of its upkeep would have far outweighed the cost of paying the Private Sector to hire out their facilities and employees to deal with this crisis.

In point of fact the NHS could have used their superfluous infrastructure to build all manner of economic buffers which, when the chips were down, they could repurpose for healthcare.

For example, the site of a derelict hospital could be redeveloped as a hotel, and run as a profit making business for the NHS, until such time as its accommodation might be needed to provide space for patients.

In this way the NHS would effectively be leasing their property to the Private Sector on the proviso that it could be reclaimed for NHS use as and when the necessity arose.

The 1945-1951 Labour Government did in fact use derelict hospital sites to build social housing, only for subsequent Tory Administrations to sell these houses off to the Private Sector.

The 1665 Plague and the 2020 Pandemic

These were two very different types of contagion, but there were many similarities in the way in which these epidemics were handled.

In 1665 it took about four months for those in charge to realise that they were not dealing with another sporadic outbreak of the Plague, but something far more potentially catastrophic.

In May 1665 King Charles and his retinue left for Oxford, and that was shortly followed by the exodos of the Upper Classes along with their servants and valuables.

The wealthy merchants of London closed down their manufacturing businesses, and withdrew from international trading, thereby leaving a vast swathe of employees without any source of income.

By July the increasing numbers of deaths, prompted the Lord Mayor of London and the administrative machinery to reinvoke the provisions provided by the 1603 Parliamentary Act, which allowed the restraining and confining of activities of London's population. This involved the closure of all places of public entertainment and hostelries, the confinement of infected people to their own homes, and the appointment of Officers to police these measures.

With so many people out of work and in need of a source of income, these dangerous jobs (buriers or sextants, carters, watchmen, nurses, investigators, etc) which all involved contact with infected people, were quickly filled and refilled when those previously employed fell ill and died.

Confining infected people to their own homes (along with their uninfected relatives and servants) merely served to wipe out whole families, OR encourage those, who realised what was happening, to escape from their watchmen and try to find somewhere outside of the city to take their dependants, and inadvertently spread the contagion.

The safest places were the hundreds of merchant ships moored in the centre of the Thames. They were inaccessible to the investigators and, where they had been under-provisioned, they could rely on safe watermen to bring them fresh food and water.

What the city needed at that time were separate places to quarantine the infected and their 'uninfected' contacts, but there was only one pest house, and it had insufficient capacity to take all the infected individuals, and nowhere to quarantine their contacts. The solution, namely the shutting up of houses, just exacerbated the situation, and the people who fared worst were those at the bottom of the capitalist human pyramid.

Treatment of the diseased, and prophylaxis for others, relied 99% of the time on unproven alchemy and barbaric medical practices, but the use of face masks, impregnated with vinegar, was adopted.

In 2020, with a vast database of knowledge at our fingertips, although no specific knowledge about how this new virus was spread or replicated, we were still unable to contain the Coronavirus, and our attempts at treatment lacked the scientific proof of efficacy. We were just lucky that this Coronavirus, despite having an enormous capacity to spread, was infinitely less virulent than the Plague!

Having lost most of our infectious diseases units, and all but demolished the ability of Public Health to deal with such an emergency, the NHS became a disaster waiting to happen.

Where had all the in-house laboratories and their staff gone? They had gone away to distant pathology hubs run by private contractors!

When it came down to the Government setting an example to the people on how to behave, MPs rarely wore face masks either in public or in the Houses of Parliament!

Self-isolation of those with respiratory tract symptoms might have been worthwhile if this had been backed up by a positive Covid-19 test, but that was a long time coming, and in the interim this created serious shortages of hospital staff.

Underlying all this was a lack of proven scientific data able to show how the virus gains entry into the body, and where it is replicated before the patient becomes a transmitter of Covid-19.

The 'experts' focussed their attention on the high-tech world of genome analysis, and ignored the possibility that the disease could, amongst other possibilities, be spread by Covid-19 contaminated food!

The Covid-19 tests were too sensitive to be able to distinguish between those who had upper respiratory tracts contaminated with Covid-19, and those who were actively replicating and transmitting the virus. This apparent inability to quantify the viral load resulted in the quarantining of people who posed no health hazard.

The belief that a vaccine would solve the problem was just wishful thinking, and a potential windfall for the pharmaceutical industry, but the problem for the vaccine manufacturer was that the viral genetic material is protected, just like the flu virus, by an envelope, which shares many features of the plasma membrane of its latest infected host cell. Picking out one part of that membrane which contained that special 'spike protein' might not be enough to confer lasting immunity, and that is exactly how it has turned out. These partially immunised individuals then merely became the vectors of the disease, and any new variants that arose as a result of natural selection.

What we really needed was something, in addition to wearing a face mask, which would prevent the virus from latching onto the host cell in the first place.

Many academic questions to answer, but nobody willing to do the research for fear that a revelation might upset those at the top of the hierarchical 'scientific' tree.

What to do?

Ignore the question or pretend it has not been asked.

People in high places don't like being embarrassed.

However, no matter how much one might criticise the NHS, the staff pulled together like never before to create teamwork that had not been seen for decades. Furthermore, all sorts of other people emerged from our social framework to carry out essential unpaid work in order to keep the wheels of healthcare turning.

This has become a social revolution, but will it be enough for the healthcare professions and the politicians to bite the bullet and relaunch the NHS?

24

Continuity of Care and the EWTD

Did the electorate realise that, with every capitalist administration they voted for, they would lose one element of healthcare which they deeply cherished, i.e. continuity of care?

With the NHS being a politically driven organisation, its weakness lay in the five year term of office of whichever political party was currently in charge of the business.

The capitalist Conservative Party moved in one direction, and the socialist Labour Party usually moved the goal posts in the opposite direction.

One victim of this debacle was continuity of care.

Doctors and nurses also understood the importance of continuity of care for their patients, but politicians barely understood the importance of building a healthcare system that would be fit for purpose well beyond their own political interests. This was self-evident in the short-sighted way in which they built new hospitals.

Building a hospital with a likely shelf life of less than fifty years was little more than jerry-building, and today we are reaping the harvest of those penny-pinching politicians.

The Prime examples in East Anglia are:

> West Suffolk Hospital – Bury St Edmunds
> James Paget Hospital – Gorleston
> Queen Elizabeth Hospital – Kings Lynn
> Hinchingbrooke Hospital – Huntingdon

These were built from 1973-1983, using light-weight poor quality reinforced (aerated) concrete in the ceilings that supported the upper story floor.

Today these hospitals are relying upon costly temporary supports to prevent the ceilings from falling upon the people below. Just now the government has no immediate plans to replace these hospitals with properly constructed buildings, able to withstand the ravages of time, and address future need.

In regard to continuity of care, organisation and reorganisation agendas nibbled away at everything. Forward planning, which could barely withstand the attrition of each five year term of office, became a politicized wish list which was dumped almost as soon as the next new Parliamentarians took their seats at Westminster.

As far as patient care was concerned one might have thought that the care providers, and the medical profession in particular, would have challenged each new government directive, but since these changes in policy were invariably laced with financial bribes, the NHS evolved without the care of the patient being uppermost in the plan.

There were four major factors which allowed continuity of care to become side-lined:

1. Loss of hospital bed capacity
2. Specialisation out-trumping general internal medicine
3. A dictat to reduce inpatient length of stay
4. The European Working Time Directive (EWTD)

Taken together, this became a pernicious game of 'Pass the Patient'.

The number of hospital beds started to decline from the very beginning, as the NHS rationalized the need for inpatient care. It was widely assumed that by improving the health of the nation, the need for hospital facilities, and beds in particular, would be reduced. In fact all they were doing was shifting that threshold, when hospital facilities would be needed for the ageing population now suffering from multiple comorbidities.

In the fullness of time some specialties, such as Rheumatology and Dermatology lost all access to hospital beds. They were deemed not to require hospital beds, because Consultants in these specialities did not take part in the acute general medical duty rota.

These specialists then organized their own 'on call' rotas in order to get the associated enhancement in their remuneration, even though their 'service' was rarely more than a telephone consultation, when and if that specialist could actually be contacted!

Furthermore, as soon as junior doctors joined their preferred specialist training programme and became SpRs, enhancement in their general medical training took a back seat.

Long-stay community hospitals, where some patients had taken up 'resident' status more than a decade earlier, were carefully scrutinized by the Geriatricians, and along with the vast numbers of patients hidden away in mental institutions, these were the first to smell the fresh air and the uncertainties of semi-independent living outside the 'safety' of the institution.

The anxiety, depression and occasional terror induced by these life changing events resulted in an increased number of patients filling GP's waiting rooms and A&E Departments. This put an extra strain on the general hospital's inpatient capacity, but without any increase in the complement of hospital beds.

The Surgeons had already rationalized their minor surgical inpatient activity by moving this tranche of patients to newly built Day Surgery Units. Potentially this gave them more inpatient beds to deal with the major surgical operations from their waiting lists.

That was until the Medics, but especially the Geriatricians, filled those vacated beds with their own medical emergencies!

Finding a bed for an emergency admission became the responsibility of the Nurse Manager of the day.

During the first few years after our DGH was opened, I was able to organise my ward discharges in such a way that we always started our 'on call' day with empty beds on our ward. As time went by we found that the team which had been 'on call' during the previous night, had already filled those empty beds, leaving us nothing for our own emergency patients. Subsequently we delayed our ward discharges until the afternoon of our 'on call' day, and thereby were able to house most of our emergency patients in our own ward.

205

Our success was in part the result of my being a 'full time' Consultant, and therefore I had the time to be more proactive on our ward, whereas the other Medical Consultants, being 'part-time', usually only managed two standard ward rounds each week.

However, in spite of our 'delayed discharges' adding to our average length of stay, our team still had a lower bed occupancy than our medical colleagues. Then the Deputy Director of Nursing claimed that we did not require as many beds as our other medical colleagues, and ring-fenced six of our beds – first for ENT patients and then for clinical haematology patients!

Our reward for using fewer beds, instead of giving our nurses a welcome breather between 'on call' days, made their work even more onerous.

Instead of the hospital opening a new inpatient resource, we were being punished for being efficient!

Although each medical specialty had their own nominated unisex medical ward, unless they had enough empty beds on the morning of their rostered day 'on call', subsequent admissions over the next twenty four hours could be scattered around the hospital in an almost random fashion, and when these beds had been filled, the corridors of A&E became their temporary resting place.

This was how the post-take Safari Ward Round became the norm, when the Consultant would shepherd his available junior doctors round the hospital, starting in A&E, and then trying to ferret out those patients, located elsewhere in the hospital, which had now become his responsibility to manage.

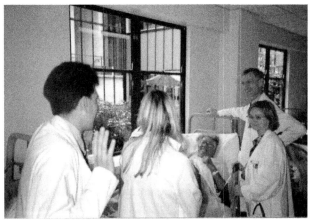

Safari Ward Round Starting in A&E Corridor

206

Reducing inpatient stay was the manager's solution to the lack of hospital beds, but it overlooked the need for more intensive GP management in the community.

Consultants were criticised by management for what appeared to them to be the excessive use of hospital beds.

Since the responsibility of each inpatient episode was laid at the door of the ultimate team which had looked after that patient prior to their discharge from hospital, our clinical skills became subverted by a game of 'Pass the Patient'.

The majority of hospital admissions were for recurrences of existing medical problems, and this led to a practice of handing back these patients, within 24 hours of readmission, to the last team which had cared for that patient, often irrespective of the specialty needs of that patient.

After the specialty of Geriatric Medicine had been established, that specialty quickly became a dumping ground for any patient over the arbitrary ageist watershed where local doctors agreed to make that division.

A common threshold for medical patients was 75.

Our Psychiatrists chose 65 to separate the young 'mad' from the elderly psycho-geriatric 'mad'.

The final nail in the Continuity of Care Coffin was the illogical introduction of the EWTD to hospital emergency care rotas.

The EWTD effectively killed off the previous team related 'on call' system, and as a result the junior doctor who admitted a particular patient stood a less than 50% chance of following up that patient's inpatient stay, and therefore was unable to learn a bit more about the natural history of disease.

What nobody appeared to realise was that if you reduce the number of hours worked then, in order to maintain the functionality of the system, you must employ more people. Managers sidestepped the issue by claiming (correctly) that there were not enough trained staff to make good the deficit. Temporary readjustments were made, but nobody bit the bullet and the need to train more staff was largely speaking ignored.

In my last years as a Hospital Consultant I would start my 'on call' day by going to the Emergency Assessment Unit (EAU), which was our combined MAU & SAU, to find out with whom I would be working. On one particular Saturday morning I discovered that the scheduled SpR had reported in sick and the Human Resources Department were trying to find a locum.

At midday a locum SpR arrived. He knew nothing about how the hospital operated and proved to be nothing more than an extra pair of hands!

Patient dissatisfaction

Lack of continuity of care doesn't have to lead to patients coming to harm or dying unnecessarily, but patient dissatisfaction can involve staff in spending hours papering over the cracks in the system, when their time could be better spent delivering healthcare.

I will illustrate this nonsensical way of managing emergency inpatient admissions with the following case history, and I will include the fallout that invariably accompanies these unfortunate affairs.

My involvement with a seventy year old patient, who had sustained a hip fracture several days earlier, only began after she had been returned from an Ipswich psychiatric unit.

During those intervening days she had been passed by the Orthopaedic Surgeons to the Geriatricians for 'Ortho-geriatric' Care.

The Indian Geriatric SHO who then saw the patient concluded, from an inappropriately carried out 'Mini Mental Score', that the patient's 'confusional state' required input from the Psychiatrists, but her opposite number pointed out that in view of the patient's age she should be referred instead to the Psycho-geriatric service.

However the local Psycho-geriatricians only looked after patients living in NE Essex, and since the patient's place of residence was just over the Essex border in Suffolk, the referral had to be made to the appropriate South Suffolk team. This unfortunate patient then found herself in a Psychiatric hospital in Ipswich.

Fortunately for the patient, the Suffolk Consultant Psychiatrist had little difficulty in realising that the patient wasn't mad, and arranged for her to be transferred back our DGH.

The medical registrar 'on call' accepted her readmission but, because it took twenty four hours to arrange transport, she actually arrived in A&E on the following day, when my team was 'on call'. Thus we became the carers for this thoroughly annoyed, disgruntled patient, who found herself once again on the Orthopaedic Ward which she had left several days earlier.

208

Smoothing over the rest of this patient's hospital stay was a herculean task, but made easier by my ward sister who agreed to have the patient transferred to a side room on our ward.

The patient was in fact a charming lady from part of a well to do family that had made their money in the furniture and aircraft industries. She had spent her early years in India and was then sent to a boarding school in England while her family remained a Delhi.

When she had come round from the anaesthetic, the first person she saw had been the female Indian Geriatric SHO, not wearing a white coat, because white coats had been considered to be intimidating, but wearing a saree instead. This saree swathed apparition reminded our patient of the Punkah Wallah's daughter with whom she had played as a young child, and it took a while for her to realise that she was not in India, but in Colchester. The doctor, who was unaware of the patient's past history, assumed that the patient was delusional, and hence the train of unfortunate consequences.

After our patient (Lady D) had been discharged with some appropriate outpatient physiotherapy to get her fully mobile again, I thought that this saga had run its course, but about six weeks later I was asked to provide a response to a complaint which had been sent in by Lady D's friend acting on her behalf.

The precise description of her miserable hospital experience cut to the quick and left no holds barred.

The procedure now was for all the staff, from the ward sisters to the lowliest junior doctors, to write a précis explaining their role in this debacle. The accumulated dossier was then fashioned into a carefully worded reply by the management's ghost writer. This was circulated to all those involved and then, once any corrections had been made, the CEO, who would not have known the patient from Adam (or Eve), nor would he have had any clinical knowledge of the problems encountered, duly signed the letter.

The impression was that the CEO had actually got involved and had personally crafted the letter himself!

That was pompous eyewash, and merely a corporate game plan that was as insincere as it was long winded.

Reassurances that, 'lessons would be learned' and that, 'remedial actions would be taken', were as empty as the promises of a political candidate seeking parliamentary election.

The letter was despatched.

Within three weeks a follow-up letter of complaint was received.

Clearly the troubled waters had not been calmed and the next phase of the complaints procedure was invoked.

This involved offering the complainant and her supporters a face to face meeting with a selection of the medical and nursing staff involved, and a group of politically motivated managers. For many complainants this could be a daunting experience, and not uncommonly the offer is declined.

209

Not so for Lady D!

The next weeks were spent finding a mutually convenient date and time for the complainant, her sponsors and all those involved.

The day duly arrived, now more than six months after the initial event, and by which time memories were fast fading into a sort of fantasy world where the facts in this case were clouded by similar past experiences and irrelevant undocumented cock-ups.

When I arrived at the meeting room, Lady D, accompanied by Maud, her friend, and a wiry balding man, with a narrow moustache and thinly rimmed circular spectacles, were already sitting at the table. The head of the table was occupied by a plump senior female administrator, who had a friendly smile set in a featureless face.

Roz, my ward sister was already sitting opposite Lady D.

There was a vacant seat next to Roz, and that gave me the reassurance of her enduring support.

I nodded towards Lady D, whispered a greeting to Roz, and sat down.

We seemed to be waiting for others to arrive.

I started to shuffle the papers which I had brought with me.

Maud whispered something to Lady D, who in turn addressed the bespectacled gentleman at her side.

One more administrator entered the room and introduced himself.

Another woman, whom I recognised as one of the hospital's ghost writers, appeared and started to offer tea and a plate of standard issue uninspiring biscuits to the assembly.

Three chairs on our side of the table remained empty.

After a long hiatus, broken intermittently by the clink of crockery and the muffled crunch of a biscuit, our chairperson cleared her throat and gave a brief preamble about the reasoning behind our meeting. The deft way in which she described the issues which we were to address made it clear that she had officiated at many such gatherings of aggrieved combatants.

From the outset there was no intention to admit to any wrongdoing, although the word 'sorry' was bandied about like some long lost part of the corporate vocabulary, but which progressively diminished in value as the frequency of its usage increased.

For her the main issue was the control of the proceedings.

For everyone else, who had read the original letter of complaint, it was the way in which Lady D had been shunted about that was at the heart of the matter. The absence from the table of anyone from either the Orthopaedic or the Geriatric Departments meant that an appropriate but embarrassing confrontation would be avoided and in its place came the carefully crafted explanations given by our politically correct chairperson.

The consummate ease with which the words tripped off her lips would have given credit to even the most accomplished public speaker.

From time to time the chairperson would hand the baton, like some illusory microphone, to either Roz or myself, for us to verbalise the excuses for the Hospital Trust's operational policies.

We had been selected because we were the last healthcare professionals who had found ourselves in charge of the patient's wellbeing.

The rules of pass the parcel (patient), made it easy to offload responsibility, unless physical harm had actually been identified, so that managerial dogma could readily supplant clinical judgement.

The demeanour of Lady D showed that she was not impressed with the politicised way in which the meeting was being conducted. She had come to confront the Punkah Wallah's daughter or failing that the Orthopaedic Consultant for whom that Indian doctor had been the clerical mouthpiece. The trail of unpleasant events had started at their behest and they should answer for their lack of care, but at every opportunity to get at the truth, the chairperson would bat the question back in the direction of either Roz or myself.

Finally, the chairperson asked Lady D if she had any further questions.

Lady D conferred with her friend and their diminutive male supporting cast, who had said nothing throughout the whole proceedings, but did not reply.

"Well then," chirruped the chairperson before any second thoughts could be mustered,

"I hope that this meeting has been helpful. We are grateful for your comments and we will make changes to our operational policies to ensure that a similar sequence of events will not happen again."

Maud took Lady D's arm and helped her to her feet.

As they walked out of the room, accompanied by the 'tea-lady', I was glad to see that she was walking pretty well, with barely any evidence of residual disability from her hip operation.

Roz and I left together. It wasn't necessary to say anything. We knew this whitewash would be a farce and so indeed it had been. The inappropriate administration of psychotropic medication to Lady D was not even alluded to. We had become part of the process of derogating ethical propriety. The voice of clinical protest had been silenced. I wondered if the matter would progress to the next stage of the complaints procedure, but thankfully nothing materialised.

Had this patient sustained physical damage, then litigation and the payment of damages might well have followed.

Lack of continuity of care has become a permanent fault line in the NHS edifice.

PART VII

Shackling the Workforce

25

Communication, IT and Confidentiality

By and large the individual medical records of patients have long been kept by the various services which each patient had attended, and these were guarded with the obsessional ownership of the banking system, so that sharing this information between different caring bodies was all but impossible.

In the early 1900s, long before the birth of the NHS, patient records held by GPs were stored in small packets called 'Lloyd George Envelopes', which were large enough to take an A5 letter folded in two. This was fine for people who remained rooted to a locality for generations, but as the opportunity to find employment further afield grew, so the need to pass on this source of medical information became more important.

In 1948, when patients had to register with a named GP, these envelopes also contained the patient's National Insurance Number – an identifier created by the need for WWII rationing cards. At this time the medical records stuffed inside these envelopes were brief notes about visits, diagnoses and treatments, and were often only decipherable by the GP, but as medical technology grew and hospital referrals became commonplace, the capacity of these envelopes to retain the associated correspondence and technological reports, became strained.

In NHS hospitals, medical records were kept in folders large enough to take an unfolded piece of A4 paper. Accordingly reports sent to GPs needed to be folded into four in order to be accommodated in the Lloyd George Envelope!

Patients, who might have been referred to more than one hospital, would then have records in at least three different places, but neither hospital nor GP had direct access to each other's records.

When computers became part of the GP practices' communication furniture, there was a need to find a way of digitising the contents of their Lloyd George Envelopes.

Information Technology (IT) companies jumped at the chance to make a quick buck and deluged the IT illiterate GPs with short sighted ways to solve the problem.

IT solutions tend to come with 'on-costs' every time the system is updated in order to improve the technology and add complexity to the record. Once hooked, the GP became hostage to this wallet massaging medium and, urged by the DoH to digitise their records, there was little time to reflect upon what was actually happening to these personal details.

Hospitals lagged behind this technological advance, mainly because the DoH was reluctant to fund digitization for secondary care, and naïve about the complexity of the issue.

The hospital record comprised of the case notes written by the medical staff. Laboratory and imaging reports were filed on separate sheets collected at the back of the file. The nursing notes, which were originally to be found in the ward register, where the senior nurse in charge penned the daily report, were then made individually and separately using a filing system such as 'Kardex'. Finally, these notes and any charts, such as TPR charts, were stuffed into the pocket at the back of the case note folder when the patient was discharged from hospital.

Patients seen in A&E had completely separate case notes, although a photocopy might be included in the patient's case note folder if the patient was subsequently admitted.

Domiciliary Care was administered in the community by District Nurses and Care Assistants, who kept their notes in a folder which was left at the patient's place of residence, so that the next carer knew what was going on. The fact that the patient, their friends and relatives could read these notes did not bother those carers, because continuity of care was paramount.

In a similar way, diabetics went on to have hand held notes.

Then there are the quasi NHS services such as Dentistry, Optometry and Podiatry with their own records which were shared with nobody!

Finally, there are the records on patients who have had private medical care, and these are not necessarily shared with anyone.

A number of half-hearted attempts were made to set up a national healthcare database, but despite vast sums of money being spent, no real progress was made.

Individuals who wanted to streamline their service developed their own IT software.

In Colchester the senior technician in the Chemical Pathology Laboratory developed a computerised system, whereby any accredited person working at the hospital could access their database via the hospital's intranet in order to see the results of patients' investigations. This was infinitely better than having to phone for a particular result or wait for the printed report to be delivered.

Likewise, I decided to computerise my Colchester outpatient clinics using 'BASIC' as the IT language.

It gave me the ability to book and change OP appointments from a remote computer and from my clinic room. In this way I could make the length of the appointment fit the clinical need, and give the patient, sitting in front of me, the ability to select a mutually convenient time for any follow up appointment.

This ran in parallel with the hospital's Patient Administration System (PAS), and this annoyed the clerical staff in outpatients to whom I gave a printout of my latest entries and amendments, for them to put on the hospital PAS.

However, my system greatly reduced the number of my patients who failed to turn up for a scheduled appointment!

There was an additional benefit in that I could write the clinic letter and email it direct to the patient's GP surgery.

This was advanced further so that my junior staff could write their inpatient discharge summaries – a significant improvement on the erstwhile handwritten often illegible discharge note.

Persuading others to use this system was not easy because they saw the existing system easier to follow, despite the inaccuracies which dogged this handwritten letter. Nonetheless it showed me just how easy a system like this could have been developed if the profession had really wanted to follow.

There was another piece of software, which I used to interrogate the PAS in order to discover where my emergencies had been admitted.

This also highlighted the fact that details on PAS had often been incorrectly entered by the clerk in A&E or the EAU.

These lowly paid employees usually had little more skill than a B&Q checkout person. Consequently the hospital had to employ a highly skilled manager to scrutinise every admission and discharge and, where necessary, correct the entry.

After I had retired I continued to provide this service, but more out of my gratitude to the coding department in whose office I had been given a *pied à terre*.

The coders used one of my printouts to discover where any uncoded case notes had gone after the patient had been discharged. Tardy coding of inpatient events earned them the wrath of the finance department, which expected the coders to massage the HRG so that the hospital could claim the maximum tariff from our PCT.

These were another group of lowly paid employees, who were expected to ferret out every possible enhancement to boost the HRG!

Unfortunately the PAS record was not fool-proof, and one particular event made me realise the pressure that A&E nursing and clerical staff were under, in order to address the 4 hour A&E discharge target.

During my daily PAS interrogation I noticed that a patient had died on Great Bentley (GBEN) ward, and was still there even though the ward had been closed for a few days, as preparation for its demolition so that the new paediatric and surgical wards could be built.

I went to A&E to dig out the patient's emergency notes, and found that on the way down the corridor he had suffered a cardiac arrest and was taken back to A&E where he had died.

The clerk, who was under pressure to get the patient officially out of A&E before the 4 hour window had expired, had accidentally entered the destination as GBEN instead of EAU (the latest place to dump A&E patients who were about to breach the 4 hour target). Until a few weeks earlier, Great Bentley ward had been that usual dumping ground for such patients and often before they were clinically stable. Since there was no clerk on Great Bentley ward to complete that particular inpatient episode, the patient's name and destination had not been removed from the PAS after he had died!

Cracking the IT problems of the NHS is absolutely essential if we were going to become more streamlined!

Throughout this nightmare of addressing safe accurate communication, nobody appeared to have considered that the patient's personal medical details should be the sole property of the patient, in much the same way that one's bank account had always been personalised and sacrosanct.

One's bank details are carefully stored by the bank and shared with nobody other than the employees of the bank who in turn are sworn to secrecy on pain of dismissal and litigation for breaching that bond of confidentiality. Access to those records and ownership in any format is in the hands of the client.

Perversely, healthcare records have become part of a collection of Curate's Eggs. For the patient to gain access to these records, the process has become convoluted and resisted wherever possible, with the glib excuse that the patient is likely not to be sufficiently qualified to understand what is written therein. Furthermore these records are but a collection of disconnected scribblings from GP files and hospital activities. Although the GP was held to be the 'guardian' of both the patient and the patient's medical record, hospitals rarely passed on a comprehensive account of every hospital attendance.

The hospital inpatient discharge notification letters are usually written by the most junior member of the team, and are rarely factually correct or more often than not illegible.

The definitive discharge summery may not follow for weeks or occasionally not at all!

During my first six months as a Medical Registrar in Glasgow, the senior Consultant dictated the discharge summary directly to his secretary.

In 2009, imagining that my medical records had been dutifully sent on to my next GP every time I changed my place of residence, I asked my GP practice in Colchester for a look at the hospital correspondence relating to two surgical procedures carried out in 1941 and 1946.

To my surprise I was informed that the GP record only went back as far as 1986!

So, have those records been destroyed, or are they filed away in some bottomless NHS pit, or was I just being fobbed off?

I only have one piece of my 'ancient' hospital history dating from 1941, when it was the Hospital Medical Superintendent who wrote the letter.

It is an excellent example of how to write a concise and accurate narrative. It had been sent to my aunt who had temporarily taken over my medical supervision.

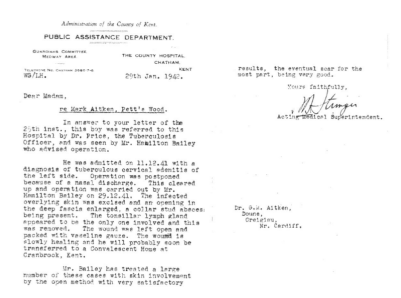

Administration of the County of Kent.

PUBLIC ASSISTANCE DEPARTMENT.

GUARDIANS COMMITTEE,
MEDWAY AREA.

THE COUNTY HOSPITAL,
CHATHAM.

TELEPHONE No. CHATHAM 3586/7-8
WS/LH.

KENT
29th Jan. 1942.

Dear Madam,

re Mark Aitken, Pett's Wood.

In answer to your letter of the 25th inst., this boy was referred to this Hospital by Dr. Price, the Tuberculosis Officer, and was seen by Mr. Hamilton Bailey who advised operation.

He was admitted on 11.12.41 with a diagnosis of tuberculous cervical adenitis of the left side. Operation was postponed because of a nasal discharge. This cleared up and operation was carried out by Mr. Hamilton Bailey on 29.12.41. The infected overlying skin was excised and an opening in the deep fascia enlarged, a collar stud abscess being present. The tonsillar lymph gland appeared to be the only one involved and this was removed. The wound was left open and packed with vaseline gauze. The wound is slowly healing and he will probably soon be transferred to a Convalescent Home at Cranbrook, Kent.

Mr. Bailey has treated a large number of these cases with skin involvement by the open method with very satisfactory

results, the eventual scar for the most part, being very good.

Yours faithfully,

Acting Medical Superintendent.

Dr. G.W. Aitken,
Doune,
Creigiau,
Nr. Cardiff.

This mess just grew as healthcare became increasingly complex, and the need for a comprehensive Electronic Patient Record (EPR) became overwhelming, but who should have access to its contents?

IT and the EPR are all about the gathering, securely storing, and ultimately the giving of accessibility to patient related data.

However, at no stage of this process was the patient's right, to have access to his or her medical information, considered.

Does any of this matter?

Clearly there needs to be a central repository of all this information and the ability of each and every patient to be able to gain comprehensive access to the data.
Most patients would not be averse to their records being perused or added to, provided that the person concerned had authorised access.

26

Pay & Conditions, Gaming and Duty of Care

If there is one way to focus the attention of a workforce which out trumps all other considerations, then it is pay and conditions, and it didn't take the medical workforce long to use this means of leverage, or the paymasters to realise how they could use this mechanism to promote their own political agendas. It all comes down to what the workforce expects to be paid for, and how the paymasters can manipulate the contracts to pay as little as possible for the work done. It also depends on whether one views the NHS as a charity or a business.

The Hospital On Call Burden
For the first four years of my life as a doctor, I accepted that working a 1:2 duty rota was par for the course. It gave great opportunity to gain experience. For the next two years as a Medical Registrar in a Glasgow teaching hospital, the rota was 1:4, but my salary was no different from my previous 1:2 rota as a Medical Registrar in England.
I suppose I saw that as a bonus. Additionally, whereas I was resident when 'on call' in England, there were no 'on call' rooms for Registrars at my Glasgow hospital, so I was basically 'on call' from home. Furthermore it was uncommon for me to have to go into the hospital on those 'on call' occasions, because the PRHOs and SHOs were far more experienced than their equivalents in England, and largely speaking they managed the 'on call' without additional help!
Inevitably a few years later, 'on call' duties became an additional payment on top of one's basic salary.

As a Senior Registrar at Barts, where we actually had to be on site when 'on call', I had to present my claim for my 'on call' duties to Professor Eric Scowen, who invariably looked at me with an element of displeasure, because he still believed that being 'on call' was still a part of one's contract!

When I became a hospital Consultant in Colchester my 'on call' commitment, which was not onerous, was part of the contract. Later 'on call' became a lever to enhance the Consultant salary, but disadvantaged Consultants, e.g. Rheumatologists, who had no hospital beds. They in turn claimed that they were permanently 'on call' and should have their salaries increased on a par with Consultants who really were part of the 'on call' rota! This caused more jockeying for position and claims for enhanced remuneration.

As for Junior Doctors, the Medical Colleges and the General Medical Council came to the conclusion that a junior doctor who was nominally 'on call' for 24 hours was likely to suffer from fatigue, and as a result might make decisions about patient management which could endanger the patient's safety.

This concept had in part come from claims of negligence, where the defence of the doctor in question had blamed the onerous nature of the duty rota rather than, ignorance, carelessness, lack of Consultant supervision, or being psychologically unfit for acute medical practice. This was solved by the introduction of the EWTD to junior doctor rotas, but at the expense of continuity of care and the associated learning experience.

The General Practice 'On Call' Burden
In General Practice, and before 1948, being 'on call' was an expected component of one's job as a GP. Patients and their relatives were mindful not to call the doctor unnecessarily because, amongst other considerations, they had to pay for it.

My aunt was a singlehanded GP in a small rural village near Cardiff. She also had her own dispensary. Being singlehanded meant that she was 'on call' 24/7, except for two weeks every summer when she employed a locum.

Her day started with morning surgery, followed by the preparation and dispensing of medications. The afternoons were spent doing surgeries at nearby villages, home visits and seeing those patients who had been admitted to the hospital in Llantrisant. The rest of the day was 'free' apart from all the paperwork and the fielding of calls.

With the creation of the NHS, although attending the doctor's surgery or calling the doctor for help was free, initially most patients respected their GP's right to have some family time. However, over time the burden of having to provide a 24/7 service to their patients without being rewarded for the associated unsociable hours of work, became the thin end of a medico-political wedge.

It had been assumed that the capitation fee covered 'on call' duties, but this additional workload could differ widely depending on where the practice was located.

In the leafy stockbroker-belt of Surrey, where the majority of the population had some sort of private medical insurance, life in general practice could be quite laid back.

In an inner city area, where poverty and social deprivation were rife, a GP's life could be far busier than that of the comfortable Surrey GP, but the capitation fee was the same.

One might have argued that since hourly paid workers were paid 'time and a half' for additional hours worked outside their contracted hours, and 'double time' for additional hours worked at night, weekends or public holidays, then the same rates should apply to doctors. However, since some of our 'on call' hours might have been spent in bed, there was no way of resolving our plight.

Those responsible for determining this component of a GP's earnings failed to realise the difference between being 'on call' in a hospital and being 'on call' in general practice.

Being 'on call' 1:4 in hospital, involved about 72 hours/week.

Being 'on call' 1:5 as a GP, involved working a similar number of hours, assuming a 08.00 – 17.00 weekday commitment, but whereas the hospital doctor worked his 'on call' with supporting staff and resources, the GP worked alone with his resources in his medical bag, while taking on huge personal responsibilities.

Remuneration for being 'on call' as a GP, should have reflected these differences. Many Practices lessened this burden by sharing this work with other practices or by using a deputising service. In that regard an allowance was added to the capitation fee which paid for the Practice to use these facilities or keep the money, but if they opted out, then 5% of the capitation fee was deducted,

In 2014, the introduction of the '111 Service' to replace 'NHS Direct', (which could be more than 100 miles from the patient's GP surgery), was supposed to relieve pressure on GPs, but for many patients, being interrogated using a tick box questionnaire, was an annoying waste of time, particularly when they were ultimately referred on to A&E or the Ambulance Service.

Over time the capitation fee became known as the Global Sum Payment (GSP) which included all sorts of adjustments, e.g. rewards for GPs if they achieved >150 points under the Quality and Outcomes Framework (QOF).

Extra-contractual Emoluments for Hospital Doctors

Paying doctors for specific services rendered had been one of the major stumbling blocks which had taxed the patience of Nye Bevan. The final agreement with the medical profession was complicated by how medical doctors with university appointments in Teaching Hospitals should be rewarded, in order to bring their salaries into line with those working in the sticks.

Bevan had already agreed that Consultants could continue to indulge in Private Practice alongside their NHS employment contract, but not all academics had the opportunity to see and treat private patients.

The solution was quite simple – pay academics enough to bring their university pay up to the equivalent of a consultant on a full-time NHS salary.

This pay enhancement was eventually called a 'Merit Award'.

However, life in the medical profession was never going to be that simple, because there were Consultants with part-time appointments at Teaching Hospitals, who also had NHS appointments at hospitals in the sticks and additionally indulged in a 'bit of Private Practice'. In fact it was this group of Consultants who put the cat amongst the pigeons, because colleagues working at the same hospital in the sticks felt that they provided educational support for their junior staff, but received no financial reward for their efforts!

Eventually the scheme of Merit Awards was rolled out into the greater NHS, but the allocation of these awards was secretive and seemed to depend upon who you knew rather than what the individual contributed to the NHS, over and above their contractual requirements.

Over the next seven decades, Merit Awards acquired different nomenclatures, and different ways of granting them. By the time Hospital Trusts had been invented, these pay enhancements were awarded by the Hospital Board, and there was a limit on the number of awards in force at any one time. At no point was an award withdrawn because the incumbent had stopped performing a particular function in recognition of which the award had originally been given!

The money shelled out on these awards came out of the overall hospital budget, and arguably that money would have been better spent on patient services.

The kudos that a Consultant gained for giving services over and above their contractual requirements should have been enough, but it looked as though we wanted both kudos and gold!

In General Practice some doctors argued that they should be included in this meritorious gravy train, although they had other ways to massage their salary without having to indulge in this particular money grubbing activity.

Extra-contractual Emoluments for GPs

Before 1948, doctors competed with each other in order to gain their share of those patients seeking medical advice and treatment. Because doctors were prohibited from advertising their skills, word of mouth was usually enough to secure a reasonable living.

General practitioners knew the expertise of those from their erstwhile teaching hospitals, so that the grapevine referral system for specialist advice became a reliable network by which a Medical Consultant could prosper and compete effectively with colleagues from the same specialty.

Likewise, in the local community, word of mouth established which GP Practices were the most sought after.

After the NHS became law, GPs acquired a flock of potential patients and an associated guaranteed income, without any consideration of how to deal with any sudden demand from numbers of people whom they had never seen before.

The more forward thinking GPs decided to form group practices, and thereby share the burden of sudden surges in demand, but also give them the means by which they could share the workload at night and weekends.

This gave GPs their first chance to enjoy some family time without the threat of disruption at any time of day or night whenever someone on their list telephoned for assistance.

Additional services such as doing one's own dispensing or the performing of minor operations were add-ons to the practice's income, and in time this became the Government's way to introduce politicised targets as financial incentives. These QOFs such as performing health checks, taking a patient's blood pressure or having the serum cholesterol measured, massaged the surgery's GSP, but involved a lot of additional paperwork.

Unsurprisingly this led to non-essential appointments filling the available appointment slots and prolonging the waiting time for more urgent appointments. Little wonder that many patients preferred to join the chaos of the nearest A&E Department, and get their problem sorted out within a few hours, as opposed to having to wait for several days or even weeks to see their GP!

Every day my GP surgery waiting room flagged up the number of patients who did not attend their appointments. Typically this varied around 200 per month. Did they not realise that if a patient has to wait days or weeks to get a problem sorted out, then the problem might have been resolved in the interim? Therefore waiting on the phone for ages to cancel that appointment then becomes a waste of the patient's time, so why bother to cancel it?

GP screening activities were claimed to reduce cardiovascular disease and increase longevity, but at the expense of side effects from drugs, the manufacture of which boosted Big Pharma and escalated NHS spending.

Blood pressure is not a disease!
It is a physiological variable which responds to a variety of homeostatic stimuli, such as posture.
The lying BP is lower than the standing BP, and the sitting BP occupies an intermediary position.
How many GPs measure the BP with the patient lying down, when this will add precious time to the appointment?
If the blood pressure is recorded as being higher than an arbitrarily defined value then, after eliminating potential, mainly endocrine causes, the condition is defined as 'Essential Hypertension', but that still does not justify medication.

There was no consideration of the real needs of patients caused by slavishly achieving Government targets.

Moonlighting
Working as a locum, outside one's contractual commitments, was one way of earning a bit more on the side.
Many nurses, who had registered with locum agencies. took on extra shifts in this way, even though this might make them less fresh and able to cope with their contractual duties.
Likewise registered doctors of all grades, who also had NHS contracts, could offer their services to locum agencies.

When I was a Senior Registrar, I worked as a locum Consultant on the Isle of Wight for two weeks of my annual holiday (with pay).

Holidays with pay had been something which the unions had fought hard for. These holidays were intended for rest and recuperation and not for a 'busman's holiday'!

229

One might consider Private Practice to be a type of moonlighting, except that it was allowed for as part of a doctor's NHS contract.

Pilfering

Being public servants and being paid out of the public purse, added one further temptation to those travelling in the NHS gravy train, but it wasn't confined to the medical profession. Pilfering from one's employer was even thought of as a rite of passage in many businesses. During my forty years working for the NHS I didn't buy a single ball point pen. Many were gifts from drug reps, but most were just there for the 'borrowing'!

My first four years as a junior doctor were spent living in hospital accommodation with the cost of full board and lodging being deducted from one's pay. We really lacked for nothing to sustain us during our long hours of work, apart from alcohol and entertainment, although absolute alcohol from the laboratory could be made into a drinkable cocktail, and nurses were not averse to attending our parties.

After completing the morning ward round, one of the perks was to sit in the ward sister's office for a cup of coffee and a bacon or scrambled egg sandwich, but on one particular morning we were told that due to a shortage of bread and milk we would have to go without! This 'shortage' persisted for several days before we heard that, when leaving the hospital after their night shift, the bags of some members of staff had been searched at the porters lodge and found to contain a variety of items which had been intended for the patients' breakfast.

However, maybe we weren't much better in so far as we were eating the bread, eggs, bacon, butter and milk left over from the patients' breakfast, but we never considered such pilfering to be in any way wrong, because we were after all paying for full board and lodging!

Some people even stooped to stealing loo rolls, even though their absorbent ability was minimal and 'GOVERNMENT PROPERTY' was stamped on each sheet.

Years later this petty thieving sometimes took on a different dimension when surgical equipment and disposable items turned up in Consultant's bags on their way to a private assignment.

The glib excuse offered for this practice was that patients treated in the Private Sector indirectly saved the NHS and the taxpayer money, and that was true!

I am not sure that we really cared that much about how this misappropriation of NHS property might affect the care of patients in the long-term.

Making a bit on the Side

At least one of our local GPs had a profitable little business importing medicines from France.

The wheeze involved taking his shooting-brake across the English Channel to France, where he purchased some crates of wine and a large quantity of commonly prescribed antibiotics and analgesic preparations.

The medicines were subsequently dispensed to his patients by his Practice Pharmacist, and the going rate for the NHS equivalent preparations recouped from the DoH.

There was nothing really illegal about this, in so far as he had saved money by cutting out their usual wholesalers and their on costs from the transaction, and paid himself for his efforts.

However, this did highlight the fact that the wholesalers of medicines must have been taking the NHS to the cleaners, if the same drugs could be bought in France more cheaply, and the GP could still make a profit on the transaction in spite of having the cost of transport and having to exchange £s for €s.

Patients were at first bemused by the wording on the packets being in French, but the Pharmacist gave them the necessary instructions in English.

27

Competition Coercion and Clinical Outcome

In the capitalist world of big business, the success of your company is all about out-competing your competitors. If your product is too pricey you will lose your clientele, even if you claim that the quality of your product is better than that of its rivals. Reducing the cost of production, by manufacturing more of the same product, might help you to undercut your rivals, but you are only likely to achieve that either by relocating your business to a country where the cost of labour is minimal, or by mechanising your production process. The latter requires extra capital and the need to borrow money to buy and install the new machinery. Once you start to borrow money to keep your business alive, you will have an extra cost pressure – paying back the loan. Alternatively you could make your company a Public Limited Company (PLC) by issuing shares, but that could bankrupt the business if profits fail to meet your investors' expectations and the investors ditch your shares. In that scenario your only salvation would be to advertise your business using false information.

Competition has no place in nationalised healthcare. The NHS has a captive market and therefore does not need to compete. Your product, namely a good outcome for your patient, depends on the infrastructure and the number and the skills of the carers. The more you invest in infrastructure, workforce and skills, the better the outcome. Streamlining the process by adopting best practice relies upon sharing your good experiences with everyone, no matter where their service is located, and not by trying to out-compete them.

However, the 2012 HSC Act created a pernicious system whereby the NHS was now **forced** to use the Private Sector, unless its own chosen service provision was less expensive.

In effect the Private Sector had been offered the opportunity to outbid the NHS for services, which the NHS had no need to put up for sale.

Joint replacement surgery was a prime target.

However, the Private Sector was not interested in taking on any patients, where risk factors could complicate the procedure or prolong the patient's hospital stay.

The NHS cost of surgery included an allowance for those patients where the hospital stay was likely to be complicated by the patient's comorbidities.

Allowing the Private Sector to cherry-pick the 'easy' stuff from the NHS menu, has the effect of increasing the unit cost of NHS procedures.

The Private Sector showed no interest in taking on the highly risky services of A&E, or emergencies in general, and where emergencies arose in Private Hospitals, it was all too easy to transfer the patient to the nearest NHS hospital, unless the managers believed that such action might tarnish their reputation or compromise their profitability.

With CCGs having to put virtually all their services out to tender, there was now an extra managerial cost to bear, and with their NHSE budget being frozen and heading for a year on year reduction, it meant that there would be less to spend on the care of patients.

The provision of community services for patients with diabetes was a prime example of how not to manage a complex medical problem, where the outcome could be driven by selecting the data and then massaging it by statistical manipulation.

Diabetes had long been a hot potato in NE Essex. Previously the AHA had tried to embarrass the hospital with bogus statistics, and eventually the PCT decided to press for the appointment of a Diabetologist. The remit of the appointee was to enhance the care of diabetics in the community. However, when the CCG took on the role of procuring services for patients, diabetic care in the community became one of their targets. This was spurred on by the claim that diabetics in NE Essex had a higher prevalence of blindness and a higher than average amputation rate. In support of this contention they had used the national HES database for 2007-2010, but this data could be interpreted in any way one wanted to in order to support one's argument!

Basically it showed that NE Essex had the second highest limb amputation 'rate/1000' (3.95), than any of the other PCTs in East Anglia, and the seventh highest rate in the whole of England. Peterborough's higher total amputation rate (4.58) was because they had far more minor amputations and therefore a lower major limb amputation rate (1.45) than NE Essex (1.63). This then becomes a grey zone in the data whereby the definition of major and minor might be interpreted differently.

Exactly the same problem arises in the definition of major and minor road traffic accidents, when it comes to deciding which parts of our road network requires re-engineering!

There was another statistic which showed that NE Essex (0.17) was only second to Dorset (0.20) in its amputation rate in non-diabetic patients.

Many people examining these data might assume that the amputation rate refers to the number of patients, but many patients were likely to have had more than one amputation during the study. Since intervention to reduce the amputation rate will be aimed at the patient and the control of their blood glucose levels, the numerator in these studies should have been the number of 'amputees/1,000' of the local population and not the number of 'amputations/1,000' of the local population.

The other interesting statistic was that there was a highly significant positive relationship between major and minor limb amputations in this cohort of 158 regions. The inference was that ischaemic vascular disease (poor blood supply) was an

235

important driving factor in regard to the risk for major limb amputations in patients with diabetes.

In the light of these statistics I went back to a similar audit in NE Essex, which I had conducted from 1992-1994 (which was before our Diabetologist was appointed).
In those 2 years there had been 204 limb amputations of which 86 had been performed on diabetic patients, and 118 on non-diabetic patients.

Statistics
The problem with statistics is that useful inferences can only be made if the data collected in different localities is truly comparable. In regard to the 2007-2010 study, how many amputations were excluded from that analysis?
This is best addressed by looking at the data collected in NE Essex from 1992-1994, where I was able to look at all the clinical details relating to each patient episode.
The first consideration was that there were 11 upper limb amputations, and of these 9 were in non-diabetics with the reason for amputation being trauma, deformity or ischaemia. In regions where upper limb amputations had not been included in their returns, that would reduce their 'rate' by about 5%.
At the time of my audit it seemed reasonable to me to exclude these from further consideration, because prevention of amputations of the lower limbs was the most important outcome to address.
Having excluded those patients, we are left with 193 amputations of which 84 were in people with diabetes and 109 without diabetes, but can we be certain that the non-diabetics did not have diabetes, because random blood glucose levels were not measured on 27 patients and 17 had a random blood glucose of >=8mmol/l.
If we exclude these 44 patients from the non-diabetic data, we are left with 129 amputations of which 84 were in people with diabetes and 65 without diabetes.

Basically it means that in our 1992-1994 data, 75 could not be accurately classified.

What about the national data collected from 2007-2010? Was the coding accurate and how many episodes were misclassified? Next, there was a misprint in the 2007-2010 report – the ratios were probably based on populations of 10,000 in diabetics and 1,000 in non-diabetics!

If 1,000 had applied to diabetics, then it would have meant that in NE Essex (population of c 300,000) we were performing more than one amputation every day, and that never happened!

Allowing for that error, one can calculate the actual number of amputations in NE Essex during those periods, and that would give an average annual number of amputations as follows:

	DIABETIC		NON-DIABETIC	
	Major	Minor	Major	Minor
1992-1994	22.5	19.5	23	9.5
2007-2010	16.3	23.2	12	6

Clearly there had been a reduction in major amputations in diabetic patients.

Does that mean that the system in force **was** effective?

So,

'If it ain't broke, why mend it'.

But our CCG overlooked these considerations, and awarded the contract to a Suffolk based consortium.

Who were the losers?

Less money would be available for other patients in NE Essex.

Local GPs might miss out on their QOF payments.

Our hospital might lose income.

Maybe the CCG had expected a better return on the PCT's original investment, i.e. the appointment of a Diabetologist.

237

As you can see, the overall effect of outside competition on medical services can be counterproductive.

In regard to these data there is an important confounding fact.

Stents and femoro-popliteal arterial bypass grafts were introduced during this interval and played an increasing part. Hence the lower amputation rate in non-diabetics, but these techniques were much less effective in patients with diabetes.

Medical statistics are a can of worms, because there are usually too many confounding variables, and they can be manipulated in whatever way the auditors wish to influence future activity or the spending on resources.

In regard to the real outcome, the removal of a few small toes only has a temporary effect on a patient's mobility, but the removal of the great toe or a mid-tarsal amputation (considered to be a minor amputation) will have lasting effects on mobility.

The **outcome** for the individual patient is their mobility, and not what the surgeons have done to their lower limbs!

In the case of the Coronavirus pandemic, we were regularly bombarded with the number of people who tested positive for Covid-19, but this is meaningless without knowing how many people were actually tested. Furthermore even that statistic tells us little about our chances of catching the disease, because a positive Covid test can't distinguish between a person whose respiratory passages are just contaminated and someone who is actively replicating and disseminating the virus!

Statistics also drove the target setting agenda of the politicians.

When the government set performance targets which also determined the level of remuneration, the temptation to fiddle the figures became a secret reality. The notion, that hospitals could do better if they pulled their fingers out, and became more efficient, was typical of the ignorant politicians who set the targets. It didn't seem to dawn on those whip crackers that in order to get better throughput, the hospitals would need investment in infrastructure, technology and staff.

The targets became the big stick and, provided that employees kept stumm, the ministers could turn a blind eye to what many of them suspected was the truth.

The most commonly fudged waiting time was the time taken from arrival in A&E to the decision to treat or discharge the patient. However, there were more serious misdemeanours which affected the quality of care, morbidity and mortality.

The target fiddling and deteriorating quality or care in Mid Staffs remained hidden from view until a member of the public opened their can of worms.

In Colchester it was a brave member of staff who chose to risk losing his livelihood, and expose the way in which cancer waiting times were being massaged.

This should have become a criminal investigation, but instead a medical based investigative team was sent to set up a series of confidential interviews with staff. This posed a considerable headache for the medical director, who was also the Caldicott Guardian, and whose task was to guarantee patient confidentiality. However for the purposes of this investigation, it was deemed essential to let the visiting team have comprehensive access to all patient related data.

The final report showed how members of staff had been cajoled into delaying the entry of patients onto the waiting list, and removing patients from the waiting list when the deadline for starting treatment was close. The report also highlighted a shortage of staff and the facilities required to complete preliminary investigations.

The hospital finished up being put into 'Special Measures' with 'experts' being parachuted onto the Board of Directors, and the CQC being given the opportunity to bleat and write threatening reports which kept the hospital in 'Special Measures' for the next five years.

Our GCE did the honourable thing and fell on his sword, but our SIC tenaciously clung on to her post, when it was probably her bullying culture which had inhibited those who could have averted this disaster and get the problem sorted out in house long before the sword of Damocles actually fell.

Statistics need to be treated with great caution, because one rarely knows the real motive of the statistic disseminator.

Was giving us the number of positive Covid-19 tests aimed at frightening the public into getting two or more vaccinations?

With diabetics, was failing to achieve 'normal' blood glucose levels intended to frighten them with the prospect of blindness, renal failure and limb amputation?

People are motivated in many different ways.
One can take a horse to water but one can't make it drink!
Just remember: '**there are lies, damn lies and statistics**'!

28

Public or Private

It has long been debated whether or where Private Practice should sit within the NHS.

All patients have the same basic anatomy and physiology irrespective of whether they want to be treated privately, just as doctors, nurses and dentists have the same basic training and develop the same skills which do not have a special programme for those who wish to practice in the Private Sector.

Basically, what the private patient craves is privacy. They do not want to be seen in the public arena alongside the *hoi polloi*, and they are prepared to pay for this privilege, although for dentistry, where dignity and privacy are enshrined in the service, it is being able to be seen without having to wait unnecessarily.

That leverage given to dentists played a minor role in the first few years of the NHS, because with the demand for dental treatment suddenly taking off, and a generous tariff for NHS dental work, dentists began to make a lot of money. However, in order to curb demand, the tariff was changed and only part of the cost of treatment was underwritten by the NHS, with the remainder paid for by the patient.

As dentistry became less profitable, dentists curtailed their NHS lists and spent increasingly more time seeing private patients.

A few years before the Covid pandemic struck, the dentist, whom I had been seeing for several decades, decided that she would in future only see private patients. I found myself at the same dental practice, but now seeing a newly recruited dentist. She was competent but not too keen to maintain the many crowns which her predecessor had inserted.

Soon after Covid struck, I developed an abscess around one of these damaged crowns. Getting an urgent appointment took time and, when the emergency was eventually treated on the NHS, there was no follow up or inclination to take on any remedial work.

Fortunately I managed despite losing fillings and another crown.

Then in July 2021 I received a call inviting me to have a routine check, but the first appointment offered wasn't until March 2022!

I took the appointment, more in hope than conviction that nothing of importance would intervene.

Two months later I received an email from the Dental Surgery which stated that in view of their limited number of NHS slots, I could avail myself of one of their unbooked private slots if I wanted to be seen sooner than March.

Hospital Consultants were not quite so unashamedly blatant about what they had been doing since 1948, but were clearly tarred with the same brush.

Outside the NHS, doctors, dentists and nurses have always been free to administer to private patients, but should they also be allowed to have NHS contracts?

This was the basic sticking point which Nye Bevan had to compromise over at the inception of the NHS. It ended up with the medical profession being given *carte blanche* to do whatever they liked, and enjoy the security of an NHS contract alongside being able to feed at the private trough! Inevitably this lead to a conflict of interests, with the ability to lengthen their NHS waiting lists and thereby fuel their Private Practice with patients who felt that they could not wait an unacceptable time to be seen or treated.

The NHS Hospital Consultant Contract rewards us with a good guaranteed salary and regular increments, six weeks of annual leave with pay, a generous pension, an entitlement to adequate study leave and a 'job for life'.

Why would anyone in their right mind give up a proportion of this in order to engage in Private Practice?

Simply, it is all about personal ego.

If a NHS Hospital Consultant wants to live in the most prestigious part of town, mix with the great and the good and run an expensive motor car, then his NHS salary and all its perks would usually be insufficient to support such a way of life, but the potential financial benefit of giving up part of one's NHS Contract, and replacing it with a lucrative Private Practice, does make good financial sense. However, in the process the Consultant becomes like the man in the fairy story who had lost his shadow. Inevitably sooner or later there will be conflicts of interest.

One cannot be the servant of two masters.

In the NHS hospital scenario, attempting to deliver care to both private and NHS patients in the same facility does not work.

When I was a surgical PRHO, the private wing at the King Edward VII Hospital in Windsor was set in the corridor next to the female orthopaedic ward, in the days before hip fractures had become commonplace..

The nurses had to service the patients in the public ward as well as those along the corridor in the private rooms, and the latter were for ever ringing their bells for attention. The ward sister had an impossible task to keep the private patients happy whilst making sure that the NHS patients were not short changed. Furthermore she was continually being pestered by the non-orthopaedic consultants to book rooms for their patients.

Then there is the question whether or not private patients and doctors working in the Private Sector should have access to NHS facilities?

In my own opinion, NHS patients should have priority to all NHS facilities and not be obliged to wait while a private patient is being seen or treated.

There is also a fundamental challenge to a doctor's conscience when posed with having to make a choice between his NHS duties and the demands of a private patient.

Having been appointed as Consultant Physician in Colchester, and having decided not to indulge in Private Practice, I found my conscience challenged when a colleague asked if I would stand in for him in regard to a patient under his care in the Private Hospital. At the time I could not find a reasonable excuse to avoid helping this colleague and, with his generous offer to pay me for my troubles, I agreed.

The task was simple. Visit the patient every day at my own convenience and, when necessary, make adjustments to his management.

This was money for old rope!

245

When asked on a second occasion to perform the same function for another of this Consultant's private patients, I agreed without giving the matter further thought.

However, whilst I was in the middle of my outpatient session at ECH, I received an urgent call from the sister at the Private Hospital, saying that the patient in question had 'collapsed'.

Without further ado, I offered my excuses to the nurse running my clinic and left her to pacify the patients waiting to see me, while I drove off down the road to the Private Hospital.

By the time I arrived, the 'collapsed' patient had partly recovered.

After examining the patient, performing an ECG, making some adjustments to the patient's medication and given the patient and his wife (who happened to be visiting) my reassurances, I returned to ECH to resume my clinic.

On reflection, although nobody had come to any harm, I had inconvenienced my NHS patients and the staff at ECH, in pursuit of personal financial gain. Clearly one cannot be the servant of two masters, and yet my colleagues who engage in Private Practice must face similar conflicts of interest on a regular basis.

This was the last time that I put myself in such an invidious position. However, in the 1990s the Consultant Contract of Full Time NHS Consultants was changed, and allowed those Consultants to engage in Private Practice, provided that their earnings from that source did not exceed 10% of their NHS salary!

This sort of moonlighting was thereby wholeheartedly approved of!

In the following case, the issues involved were much more complex, and that was not just because the patient died after what should have been a straight forward surgical operation.

The patient (Mr X) was a retired 66 year old Northern Irish builder, who had decided to get a knee replacement performed by Mr A at the Clementine Churchill Hospital (CCH), a Private Hospital in West London. Mr A was a very experienced Orthopaedic Surgeon, who had successfully performed this sort of operation on a large number of patients.

On 6th February 2010 Mr X underwent total knee replacement without suffering any apparent intraoperative complications, but on the 5th postoperative day Mr A was concerned that Mr X had developed severe abdominal pain, and contacted Mr B, a colorectal surgeon, who at that time was performing his NHS duties at a nearby West London Hospital.

Mr B travelled to the CCH and saw Mr X at around 21.00 hr, when it was apparent to him that there was clinical evidence of peritonitis and the likelihood that Mr X had a perforation of his bowel. He gave verbal instructions to the Resident Medical Officer (RMO) and arranged for Mr X

246

to have a CT scan, in order to determine the likely site of the bowel perforation.

Mr B expected his management plan to stabilize Mr X's condition and allow him to fulfil his busy NHS schedule on the 12th February and then proceed with the definitive operation at the CCH, but there were difficulties in getting an available operating theatre and anaesthetist, and as a result the operation did not commence until 22.00hr on 12th February. He also discovered that the RMO had not prescribed the broad spectrum antibiotic therapy in accordance with his verbal instructions 24 hours earlier!

The emergency surgery proceeded and was complicated by an unexpected amount of haemorrhage. Postoperatively the patient did not regain consciousness, and died 48 hours later.

Since the death had occurred after a surgical operation, the case was automatically referred to the Coroner. He then requested depositions from the doctors involved in the case, the post mortem report and a response from the CCH.

Professor Duncan Empey, group medical director of the Churchill Hospital's parent group BMI Healthcare (formed in 1970, when US hospital group AMI acquired its first hospital in the UK), commissioned a detailed report from the CCH but, being a private company, he knew that he had no obligation to disclose all the details.

This report was delivered to the Coroner on 14th March.

In the NHS, this investigation would have been handled rather differently. Although a similar in depth investigation would have been carried out by the hospital, the final report would have been given to the Coroner without any redactions.

In the meantime Mr B was allowed to continue to practice at the CCH and his NHS hospital.

Then a doctor, from 'Healthcare Performance Ltd', was commissioned by the CCH to interview Mr B and investigate whether or not he might have been involved in similar incidents.

Their report was given to the CCH in July and in September they suspended Mr B from further clinical activities. By then the GMC had become involved and on 15th October there was a 'Fitness to Practise' hearing, but they decided in the end that there was no case to answer!

From the information available, a session of the Coroner's Court was convened on 18th October. At the hearing the Coroner started with the evidence provided by Mr B, and then decided on that evidence alone, that there was a case to answer, and that there had been some misdemeanour or wrongdoing amounting to criminal negligence and manslaughter.

The Coroner is not required to have either medical or legal qualifications. His opinion is personal and in this particular case he wanted an explanation as to why it took over twenty four hours for the seriously ill patient to be taken to the operating theatre.

The inquest was adjourned, and the case was referred to the Crown Prosecution Service (CPS), and from there a Police investigation was started. In view of this development the GMC became involved again, and in November it commissioned an expert witness to write a report, but all he had to go on was the redacted Empey Report.

The GMC decides to restrict Mr B's clinical activity, but the Medical Director at Mr B's NHS Hospital remains happy to allow him to continue to work there.

In July 2012 Mr B was charged with Manslaughter and Perjury.

He was suspended from his NHS post on 10th July without pay.

On 19th July he was suspended from the GMC register pending the result of the trial, which was set for 2nd October 2013 at the Old Bailey.

For the next fifteen months Mr B had no source of income or prospect of finding work. He had no access to either the CCH, which was busy ensuring that the hospital's reputation remained unblemished, or his NHS hospital, where all his records had been frozen. Could he be sure that the MPS (his medical protection insurance policy) would employ the best barrister to defend him and access all the relevant medical details pertaining to the case from the secretive vaults of the CCH? Would any of the legal arguments refer to the result of the PRISM study, published in the BMJ in 2012, which showed that preventable hospital deaths were usually multifactorial, were rarely the result of a single error of judgement, and that looking for a single scapegoat was counterproductive?

So, let us re-examine this case, using all the evidence which should have been available, and start at the beginning. Also let us not forget that the information volunteered by the patient has to be treated with a certain amount of caution.

How often do we find that the patient has been economical with the truth?

Why did Mr X seek out a private hospital in London for his total knee replacement? There were plenty of competent Orthopaedic Surgeons in Northern Ireland and no shortage of suitable private hospitals.

Was there something about Mr X's medical history which had already made the Northern Irish Surgeons disinclined to operate?

Was Mr X really unaware that he had chronic liver disease, and that this would add serious risks to any surgical procedure?

Did Mr A make a detailed assessment of Mr X's risk factors, and also communicate with Mr X's GP in Northern Ireland, before deciding to take on the case?

If a proper preoperative health check had been carried out either by Mr A or his anaesthetist, then pre-existing chronic liver disease would have been detected and made them extra cautious about the use of any drug which relied upon hepatic detoxification, e.g. morphine and its derivatives.

At that time it was standard practice to prescribe Dabigatran, a Thrombin antagonist, to prevent postoperative thromboembolism in patients undergoing total hip or knee replacements. The manufacturers marketed this drug for this specific purpose and promoted its use because it required no monitoring, <u>but did warn prescribers only to administer it with extreme caution in patients with liver disease</u>!

What efforts did Mr A and his anaesthetist make to exclude liver disease?

It is foolhardy to prescribe any drug if there are no means of assessing its efficacy and safety!

As far as Mr X was concerned, was he so unhappy with having to spend the rest of his life with chronic knee pain and limited mobility, that he would risk his life having that potentially curative surgical procedure?

Didn't he realise that by concealing his past medical history from his medical attendants, he would risk taking them down with him if it ended fatally?

In my experience, patients can on occasions be quite economical with the truth!

The total knee replacement operation was performed on 6th February 2010 without any apparent intraoperative complications. Postoperative treatment with Dabigatran was commenced and a regimen of postoperative pain relief was started, but what drugs for pain relief were prescribed?

NSAIDS are commonly used to reduce swelling around the operation site, but these drugs, particularly in the elderly, have one very serious potential side effect – perforation of the stomach or bowel!

When did Mr A first become aware that Mr X was suffering from abdominal discomfort? Was it really only on the fifth postoperative day?

On 11th February, when Mr A requested help from Mr B, the signs of peritonitis would have been obvious. He would have known from his training as a surgical registrar, that peritonitis carries a serious risk of death if not dealt with promptly. He also knew that the CCH was not geared up to dealing with any surgical emergency other than intraoperative emergencies, so why did he not immediately ring for an ambulance and transfer Mr X to the nearest NHS hospital?

Perhaps it was all about the culture at the CCH.

An unexpected emergency in a private hospital, requiring immediate transfer to the NHS, would have generated scrutiny from the local press, and this would have affected the reputation of the private hospital. A tarnished reputation could lead to a lack in confidence and a reduction in patient referrals, and thereby the hospital's profitability.

For private hospitals, profitability is the name of the game. By only operating on patients with negligible risk factors, the hospital's staff

249

requirements are minimal, and it is the employment of staff that is their main cost pressure.

Consultants working at private hospitals are not members of staff and do not contribute to that cost pressure, but many of them have shares in the company which owns the hospital, and therefore benefit from the hospital's profitability in addition to the fees charged to patients,.

So, why did Mr A decide not to refer Mr X to the nearest NHS hospital? Furthermore did Mr A convey the urgency of this referral to Mr B?

When Mr B came on the scene late in the evening of 11th February, he would have been well aware of the seriousness of Mr X's condition.

So why did he not send the patient straight to the nearest NHS hospital?

Maybe it was for the same reasons as Mr A, or did he think that he could be the knight in shining armour and rescue Mr X from the jaws of death without having to embarrass Mr A or the culture of the CCH? Either way it turned out to be a bad decision, because there was also the unknown hazard of Dabigatran lurking in the wings.

His decision to procrastinate could have helped in his favour, because it would have given time to stabilize the patient's condition by ordering the usual combination of 'suck and drip' and an umbrella of antibiotic cover.

He gave these instructions verbally to the RMO in much the same way that he would have done back at his NHS hospital, but by failing also to document those instructions in the patient's case notes, he gave the RMO and the CCH the opportunity to hold Mr B to account if all did not go well.

Mr B had an additional problem in so far as he had busy NHS commitments planned for 12th February. Should he cancel those commitments and give preference to his private patient, or could he operate on Mr X later that afternoon or evening, without adding any extra risks to Mr X's recovery?

So Mr B decided to order a CT scan in the hope that it would identify the site of the intestinal leak, and that in turn would help him to decide where to make the initial incision.

Back in Mr B's NHS hospital his surgical registrar would have prescribed antibiotics even if Mr B had not mentioned them, but RMOs are a completely different kettle of fish. These posts are not recognised by either the RCS or the RCP as suitable jobs for trainee doctors, and as a result these posts are usually filled by overseas doctors trying to get a foothold on the British healthcare ladder.

If push came to shove a RMO would be unlikely to admit to his own omission for fear of jeopardising his future in the NHS.

On 12th February Mr B was frustrated by his initial inability to get access to an operating theatre and an anaesthetist at the CCH. This was eventually resolved late that evening when Mr B also discovered that the antibiotics which he had ordered twenty four hours earlier had not been prescribed! He must have feared the worst when, after opening the abdomen, there was excessive bleeding – thanks to the Dabigatran!

250

Mr B's trial at the Old Bailey on 2nd October 2013, (three years and nine months after the death of Mr X), was a travesty.

No reference was made to the PRISM study, which had shown that preventable hospital deaths were usually multifactorial, and the identification of a scapegoat or fall guy was unhelpful in resolving the contributory factors. In this way the prosecution paid little or no attention to the post mortem finding of cirrhosis of the liver. The patient's pre-existing liver disease would have contraindicated the use of Dabigatran – a drug which undoubtedly caused the excessive bleeding during the abdominal surgery, and thereby contributed to the fatal outcome.

The need to keep the reputation of the CCH unsullied was easy, because the Empey report had been carefully redacted in their favour.

The jury found Mr B guilty of manslaughter, but were their members completely unbiased in regard to the obvious fact that the defendant's skin was not white?

While Mr B was serving his 30 month prison sentence, his real friends joined together and successfully had the verdict overturned and his name on the GMC register restored, but this was too late to undo the damage to Mr B's reputation.

This was a complex case and involved not only the doctor's conflict of interest but also the conflict between the public and private providers of healthcare. The public sector puts the interests of the patient first, whereas the Private Sector's prime objective is that of making a profit.

The medical profession has a serious problem to address. Should their members continue to benefit from a contract with the NHS, and also keep the goose which lays the golden eggs?

By 1950 when the dust had settled and they could see quite plainly that working for the NHS did not affect their income from Private Practice, should they not have searched their social consciences and decided to relinquish either their Private Practice or their commitment to the NHS?

They didn't, and henceforth could be seen as a profession which was open to financial blackmail by whichever political party was in the driving seat!

For the hospital Consultant, the simple solution would be to make a clear separation in regard to his activity. Doctors would have to make their minds up and opt for either working whole time in the NHS or in the Private Sector, but not working for both branches of healthcare.

If all NHS hospital Consultants were employed on full time contracts, the hospitals would have to provide more facilities and employ more staff in order to keep waiting lists at a similar level to those achieved in the Private Sector, and NHS Consultants might be expected to move between NHS hospitals in order to address shortfalls, but that is what is required.

All this would still guarantee a 'job for life' for NHS employees and a handsome pension on retirement.

PART VIII

A New Health Service

29

The Way Ahead

Having politicians leading and conducting the NHS, is like employing a deaf, dumb and blind person to lead and conduct the London Symphony Orchestra.

The weakness of the NHS Orchestra lies not only in it having an incompetent conductor, but also with the individual instrumentalists, who are neither following the score nor playing in tune.

Pure cacophony!

Unless doctors, nurses and other healthcare professionals work together as a team dedicated to the principles of the NHS, then we will continue to have today's dysfunctional health service, and nothing of any real significance will be achieved as we muddle our way forwards!

Therefore let's start by declaring the NHS bankrupt – the Coronavirus pandemic was the final straw.

The DoH should break up the NHS into four new services but still funded by the DoH:

1. English Health Service – EHS
2. Welsh Health Service – WHS
3. Scottish Health Service – SHS
4. Northern Irish Health Service – NIHS

Creditors would be compensated but with the smallest getting the lion's share. The larger creditors, such as those money chandlers who bankrolled the PFIs, would get the least – poetic justice for those who gladly took the NHS to the cleaners and now can swallow a dose of their own medicine!

In many ways this new beginning would be like what happened in 1948, when Britain had been bankrupted by WWII, but seventy or so years of having found out how not to run a national health service should help the new services to learn from those mistakes.

Consultants
New employment contracts for NHS staff would be required, but the contracts for the Consultant grade should be fulltime, and outlaw any moonlighting in Private Practice. If Consultants threatened a national walkout, then the DoH could adopt the ploy used in the 1960s when they upgraded Senior Hospital Medical Officers and some Senior Registrars to the vacant positions. Were the Medical Profession to agree to this change, it would show contrition for how we milked the system and ignored our responsibilities over the past seventy four years.

Thereafter an Act of Parliament could decree that once SpRs had completed their specialist training, their first ten years as a Hospital Consultant should be spent working full time for the NHS.

A similar suggestion was made by a minister in Tony Blair's cabinet, but then dropped when she realised that the medical profession would oppose it.

After completing their compulsory ten years of Consultant input, Consultants could then opt for going into full time employment in the Private Sector, or remain with their NHS career structure.

There is also a need to outsource some of the Consultant's technological activities, such as endoscopy, the insertion of stents, etc, to non-medically trained personnel.

General Practitioners
General Practice could follow the example shown by hospital Consultants, becoming salaried fulltime employees and able to enjoy a job for life and a generous pension without having to dance to the latest crackpot tune of the politicians. The patient's

first call for help should become the Doctors' Surgery, and not '111' or any other ridiculous quango, and with all the money spinning diversions, such as QOFs, taken from the GP's former activity, there would be ample time to see most patients on the same day.

Surgery location would be better if there was a central surgery in a health centre and satellite surgeries operating from 08.00-18.00 in more distant parts of the patch.

The Health Centre could then become the ambulatory part of Primary Care and also serve as a location for hospital outpatients and Public Health services.

Dentists
Where do Dentists fit in?

They had a very lucrative introduction to the NHS, but today there is a need to change the way they are contracted to provide their service. Making Dentists follow my proposed change in GP contract, i.e. making them fulltime NHS employees, should stop the pernicious business of them offering fast Private Practice as an answer to waiting lists and, like Hospital Consultants, they would have to choose between being fulltime NHS employees, or work in the Private Sector, with no option to moonlight or have their feet in both camps.

IT
After sorting out the staffing of the NEW NHS, the next key issue in this plan should be to develop an IT system which focusses on the patient, and with every patient being the owner of their individual patient related data. In this way any healthcare professional with the approved permission would be able to see every healthcare intervention in the individual's patient record, and add to it if they had read/write authorisation.

The patient would remain the owner of the record and have access to it, although without the ability to change any of the entries (i.e. 'read only'). Should the patient find errors in the record, then the person who had entered the incorrect data would be made duty bound to correct it. Such a database would make a massive difference to patient management, give an accurate medication history, and also reduce the number of unnecessary repetitive investigations at different NHS sites.

If virus-proof banking software can be written, then there is no reason why a specially commissioned IT company could not solve this problem and keep the data and access to the data safe. Should the patient have any say in this scheme?

In my opinion the answer should be 'no'.

Having their healthcare data on a personal database, should be conditional upon using NHS facilities, and not subject to patient choice.

Nurses

Nursing would require less in the way of restructuring, but the current vogue for making nursing a university degree requires a little more thought. Returning to the system where major hospitals had their own individual schools of nursing would in my mind be more sensible. There would be nothing to stop a girl from taking a university degree in natural sciences or sociology while she is making up her mind whether or not to devote her life to nursing.

In bygone times it was standard practice to read classics at Oxbridge before taking the plunge into the Holy See and being ordained for a life in the Church of England.

Paramedics

The other health related professions might require some modifications. For example, Paramedics would be of greater use if separated from the Ambulance Service, and instead allied to General Practice and the hospital emergency services.

Public Health

Public Health should be reborn with the remit of disease prevention, which would therefore no longer form a part of a GP's job description. The role would involve the screening for preventable diseases and immunisation programmes where vaccines are of proven long term efficacy.

The senior staff would be able to take control of epidemics and other environmental challenges

Community Centres and Hospitals
Community Centres should be built at the centre of gravity of the local population, and deliver Public Health, but also act as a venue for hospital outpatient services, and thereby free up the hospital campus to concentrate on emergency and waiting list problems.
The hospital does not need to be in the centre of town. A Greenfield site would be ideal, provided that it had good access to public transport.
The design and building of these Health Centres and Hospitals will need to be free of built in obsolescence, and the jerry builder's cashcow.
New hospital wards would be safer and better staffed if they were designed in the style of the Nightingale Ward. Single rooms were not meant for the privileged, but for the dying, the immunocompromised, the disruptive and those whose bodily odours would make life a misery for other patients if included in the general ward.
No more unisex wards!
Patient observation, and accessibility of patients to the nursing staff, was better in Nightingale Wards.
The opportunity to take on a better focussed hospital environment is here with the four structurally compromised hospitals in East Anglia, namely Hinchingbrooke Hospital, and the hospitals in Kings Lynn, Bury St Edmunds and Gorleston, where cheap aerated concrete was used in the structure separating the ground and first floors.
These new hospitals should be built to provide beds for emergencies and planned procedures, and space for the supporting departments, e.g. Pathology.
Accommodation for staff, and a proper doctors' mess, should form part of the central core.
A part of the campus, well away from the main hospital, could be built like an hotel with single room accommodation. This

could be used as an hotel and provide the NHS with some income, but be available as a quarantine facility in much the same way that the Fever Hospitals had provided isolation in the past.

Infective diseases units would be better placed either as separate buildings or at the extreme edge of the main buildings, with external access as the usual way in which staff and patients gain entry.

The prefabricated Great Bentley Ward at Colchester's DGH, which was bulldozed to make way for a new Paediatric Ward and an extra Surgical Ward, would have been ideal, being also next to the mortuary!

Outpatient facilities could then be provided in Community Centres close to the centre of the local population, and equipped with modern imaging facilities and laboratory testing opportunities.

In this way the patient's visit could become a 'one stop shop', including minor surgery not requiring general anaesthesia.

Patients identified as requiring inpatient hospital treatment and surgery could then have their pre-assessment examination here, knowing that their admission would take place soon afterwards.

Designing and supervising the building of NHS real estate should carry with it the risk of litigation and a custodial sentence where the building is found to be inadequate. Filing for insolvency should not be a way out of meeting the commitments of an NHS contract.

The new hospitals required in East Anglia to replace those which are falling apart, should offer a chance for architects and the construction industry to shine.

Litigation and Insurance
Inappropriate comments, written in the patient case records by naïve medical professionals, could open a lucrative can of worms for litigious profiteers. Medical mistakes which cause harm have long been an expensive drain on the financial

262

resources of hospitals. With a comprehensive IT system in place, the scope for aggrieved individuals to find fault and claim compensation would be likely to increase.

In Sweden, a medical practitioner, who has unintentionally offended or caused a harmful complication to a patient's outcome, apologises and freely admits to their errors and leaves his insurance company to agree on any reasonable settlement.
If we adopted their system we would avoid long periods of squabbling, and the massive expense on lawyers' fees, which compromised the previous exercise of fault finding and culprit identification. Furthermore it would readily open the door to finding safer ways of delivering healthcare.

Management
In the community the experiment using CCGs as the local distributer of DoH money worked well in NE Essex, except for the GP's perceived conflict of interest. It would be better if those in charge were elected by the local population to form what we might now call Local Clinical Groups (LCGs). They would know the health needs of their catchment population much better than any other more widely based consortium. It would need some clinically qualified members – preferably retired doctors and nurses – in order that it did not get carried away by some utopian dream.
Like the erstwhile CCGs it should have an elected public advisory group similar to our CCG's HFC, which in turn holds public meetings to gather the concerns of the local population.
The present FHT system would need some radical changes. Funding would come directly from the new type of CCG in the form of an allowance, and there would be no need for PbR.
Monitor and the CQC would need to be abolished.
Consequently the Cogwheel system of management, which worked so well until the politicians took over the reins, should be reintroduced.
The remit for the Governors' Council would also need to be reworked. In Colchester's case, members should only be elected from amongst those registered with a NE Essex GP Practice,

and in turn they would elect their own Chairman and thereby free it from coercion from the hospital's Board of Management.

The Board would require non-medical input from a Director of Finance, a Director of Human Resources and others, but there should be those with medical and nursing qualifications leading the orchestra, and in order not to create conflicts of interest, these posts might best be filled by retired senior doctors and nurses.

As with the Cogwheel system, there should be Divisional representation on a MEC, with their Chairman sitting on the Board, but the Chairman of the MAC should also have a place.

Audit

Auditing the performance of the health service in general, and hospitals in particular, needs to be ramped up.

There really is no longer any place for the CQC, whose only tool has been the big stick.

Finding out where things have gone wrong, along with the sharing of best practice between other parts of the service needs to be adopted. Mortality audits require input from outside the hospital, and retired doctors and nurses might be best placed to deliver this essential part of the service along the lines of the PRISM study.

Funding the New Service

General taxation aimed at the income and wealth of the population should be the main source of finance.

For us, the patients, there is no such thing as a free lunch.

Finding the financial resources to maintain the service should just be a matter of taxation, but we must also accept that certain procedures and treatments will be given on the basis of medical need, and not as part of a patient's wish list.

Unfortunately 'rationing of healthcare' will raise the issue of which clinical procedures are purely 'cosmetic' and therefore should not be available on the NHS.

In that case where would treatments such as artificial insemination and other fertility treatments lie?

The argument that an infertile woman's psychological health would be damaged, by denying her the ability to produce her own family, is specious. Instead she could be praised for having played a small part in the limitation of our population, which in its present uncontrolled state merely fuels the need for resources, and in turn contributes to the problem of global warming.

If there is to be, 'rationing', then these lines need to be drawn up by common consent, and not by the medical profession, the politicians or the pharmaceutical industry.

We all pay in one way or the other for the care we receive from the NHS. You might describe it as a National Health Insurance policy except that, unlike most health insurance policies, there are no almost invisible small print exclusion clauses.

The wealth of Britain and its former Empire had been built on a capitalist agenda, but the British, like those from other nations, also embraced a charitable conscience. However, nationalised charity, unconditionally financed by the wealthy, does not sit well in our culture. For the British to accept that change of direction we would have to become a socialist democracy!

However, the money must be sufficient to deliver a service which is not constrained by waiting lists, or lack of staff, hospital beds or equipment. Therefore taxation aimed at income and wealth would still be the best way to put healthcare on an even playing field, but how could the wealthy also satisfy their desire to do charitable deeds?

There is something about charity which gives the donor a warm feeling inside – a feeling that they have given assistance to an underprivileged member of the human (or animal) species. Taking away that feel-good-factor and making charity part of a nationalised organisation like the NHS, deprives us of that comfort. Furthermore it deprives us of deciding where any donation should be spent.

Since the NHS is currently funded out of general taxation, perhaps the taxpayer, and in particular the payer of income tax, should be allowed to decide the proportion of their income tax

265

which would go towards providing healthcare. The annual amount paid would then be kept in a database, accessible to the public on a FoI basis.

This concept could be extended to deciding on the proportion which should be spent on 'Defence', although the MOD is in reality a Ministry of Offence, since it supports military action beyond our shores!

Academic Medicine

We need to find a way of freeing Academic Medicine from their reliance upon Big Pharma for their funding.

A body like the MRC, receiving funding from the Treasury and charitable sources, including 'no strings attached' Big Pharma, could lead to a more focussed approach to the aetiology of disease, rather than the development of non-curative therapies.

A better understanding of the viral envelope, typical of the Coronaviruses (e.g. Covid-19 and Influenza), which shares many features of the host cell's plasma membrane, might enable us to find a way of disabling the virus before it becomes adsorbed onto the cell surface. The risk posed by vaccines is the possibility of one's antiviral antibodies co-reacting with healthy cells, and initiating what we currently describe as an 'autoimmune' disease.

Is this what we are currently describing as 'Long Covid'?

Training the Workforce

The training of doctors should be revised in view of the current ability of 'non-medical' technicians to deliver similar services.

A university degree is superfluous in regard to the role that many doctors will subsequently play. The previous qualifications of MRCS and LRCP, which were awarded by the College of Surgeons and College of Physicians respectively, would suffice. Those who started their medical careers with a university Natural Sciences degree might go on to become the future academics, and play a more important part in the advance of medical knowledge.

Many technical procedures have already been devolved to non-medically trained staff, in imaging and endoscopy.

The training of Radiographers/Ultrasonographers to accumulate the skills of a Radiologist might mean that only the head of department would need to be medically qualified. I guess that there are school leavers who would welcome such a job.

Pay and Conditions
The NHS works 24/7 and currently most members of staff make a variable contribution to working unsociable hours, i.e. at night, weekends and public holidays.
Recognising this dedication to work would be better rewarded if all members of staff were paid a salary which included this 24/7 commitment, without there having to be claims for working beyond their '9-5' contract. The salary for those members of staff unprepared for that 24/7 commitment should then be about 50% lower.

These are just some of the ways in which a reborn health service could be developed.
In 1948 there was uncertainty about whether this bold socialist experiment would work, and leave those providing the care worse off, but the latter proved to be unfounded.
In fact we have prospered at the expense of the system.
We partied while the infrastructure crumbled.
When the light at the end of the tunnel went out, we were lost.
The practise of medicine has never been straightforward, because sooner or later one is confronted by divided loyalties or conflicts of interest.
In one way or another we all lost the plot and just muddled on.
The Medical Profession, who had been given the key to a goldmine, were then reluctant to hand it back.
The politicians, who refused to give up the principles of capitalism in exchange for social reform.
The voting public, who saw self-interest as their guiding light, and failed to see through the murk of the political propaganda.

Decide for yourselves how this reincarnated health service can be moulded, and where other changes need to be made!

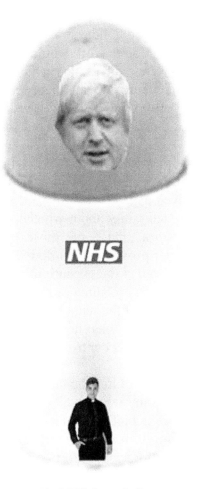

The NHS Curate's Egg

Postscript

Over time the NHS has become like the Curate's Egg.

Very good in parts!

It doesn't have to be like this.

The medical profession needs to regain the moral high ground and take back control from the politicians.

Sharing good practice and building healthcare facilities which are intended to last, should be the way forward.

When the Coronavirus Pandemic struck, the politicians had nothing left to offer us other than, '**Stay at home and protect the NHS**' whilst they really meant, '**Stay at home and protect our reputations**'.

There will be no quick fix.

Now is the time to look at how everything about the ethos of social healthcare has changed, and how we should work together to address the issues.

This is a task for everyone.

Chickening out is no longer an option.

However, before I close, here is a word of caution to all those who think they know everything, and where serendipity can save or destroy you!

Several years ago a young woman was admitted as an emergency under my care. She was unconscious and had a long psychiatric history. A simple laboratory test showed her to have water intoxication as a consequence of the inappropriate antidiuretic hormone (ADH) syndrome. Furthermore her psychiatric medication had recently been changed to lithium, and since lithium therapy can cause inappropriate ADH secretion, the diagnosis and its cause were cut and dried! She was deprived of water, and within 24 hours she had regained consciousness.

A day or so later she was discharged with advice to her Psychiatrist not to continue the lithium therapy. However within a few weeks she was readmitted when a different medical team was on call. They decided to hand her back to my team, but not before they had started an infusion of hypertonic saline. Fortunately I was able to stop the infusion before any serious damage had been done, and after a couple of days of water deprivation she was able to be discharged. To my annoyance the lithium therapy had been reinstituted by her doctor.

After this there were two more admissions, and once again she was back on lithium. I began to wonder if she was deliberately taking an excessive dose of the medication or even attempting suicide.

A discussion with her in-laws revealed that they were very annoyed with the woman's parents, who had not disclosed the girl's psychiatric history before she had married their son.

Then on one weekend, when my respiratory and infectious diseases colleague's team was on duty, this lady was admitted once more with similar symptoms but also a mild fever. Being the weekend, the patient's old case notes were not available, and the Registrar wondered if she might have meningitis. He needed to exclude raised intracranial pressure, but unfortunately he was unable to see her optic discs. That being the case, he contacted his boss who, with great difficulty, persuaded the duty Radiologist to perform a CT scan.

To the delight of the Registrar the scan revealed a tumour about the size of a golf ball sitting in her frontal cortex, and she was dispatched to our neurosurgery referral centre.

When I heard about this embarrassing situation I felt very humbled.

I had been so self-confident with my diagnosis that it had not occurred to me that there might be something else contributing to the patient's psychiatric condition or indeed the inappropriate ADH syndrome.

In fact, even her psychiatric condition alone might have been caused by this tumour, and the lithium therapy had all along been a red herring!

Had this patient's old hospital notes been available when she arrived, the tumour might never have been discovered!

Serendipity is a great leveller!

Overegging one's confidence can be a disaster.

We all need a little more humility and less hubris

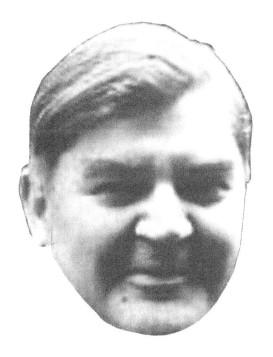

Nye Bevan, who died prematurely at the age of 62, would turn in his grave if he knew what we have done to his NHS!

Printed in Great Britain
by Amazon

42901302R00169